# Dietary Fiber: Essential To The Human Microbiome and Health

ISBN-13: 978-1545015421
ISBN-10: 1545015422

June 2018

By Peter V. Radatti

# TABLE OF CONTENTS

DISCLAIMER..................................................................5

ACKNOWLEDGEMENTS..............................................7

The cover photograph was licensed from istockphoto.com........7

Explicate permission to quote other authors are contained within the text. All trademarks are the trademarks of their respective owners........................................................7

COPYRIGHT NOTICE AND EDITIONS.............................8

PREFACE – PLEASE READ..............................................9

    Origins.........................................................................9

    The Microbiome........................................................10

    The Role of the Physician.........................................10

    Footnotes..................................................................10

    Conspiracy Theories.................................................11

    Diversity of Research Findings................................11

    A Wonder Food?......................................................12

FAIR DISCLOSURE......................................................14

I: WHAT IS DIETARY FIBER?......................................16

    Water-Insoluble Fibers............................................17

    Water-Soluble Fiber................................................21

    Soluble vs. Insoluble: Benefits.................................23

II. DEFINING DIETARY FIBER....................................23

    Understanding the Role of Dietary Fiber...............26

    What Does It Do?....................................................27

    The Bacteria Connection........................................29

    How Much Is Enough?............................................31

Suggested Dietary Fiber in Grams Per Day (g/d).................32
Quantity of Food Needed to Obtain 35 Grams/Day of Dietary Fiber..................33
The "Up" Side of Fiber.................34
The "Down" Side of Fiber.................36
Synopsis.................38

## III. THE EFFECT(S) OF DIETARY FIBER.................44
You Are Not A Human!.................46
Defination of Mitochondria from Dictionary.Com.................47

## IV. SYMBIOTES!.................49
Effects on Age, Sleep, and Circadian Rhythm.................51
Microbiome Players.................54
Combinational Benefits.................57
Food-Like Probiotic Supplements.................58
Kombucha: Benefits of a Probiotic Drink.................58
What about Parasitic Worms?.................61

## V. YOU HAVE THREE BRAINS.................63
Super Brain (3 combined).................65

## VI. REFINED SUGAR AND HFCS.................66
Role of Sugar in the Body.................67
Effects of Sugar on the Liver and Gut.................68
Biome Changes Due to Sugar.................69
How Hormones Change Due to Sugar.................70
Identification of Sugars Hidden in Foods.................71

## VII. HUMAN MICROBIOME VS. FERTILIZERS AND POISONS.................73
Chemical Poisons in the Diet.................74
Gut Bacteria: Friend Or Foe?.................77

## VIII. SPECIAL FOODS BEYOND FIBER.................78

- Slippery Elm...............78
- Honey...............79
- Slippery Elm Honey Balls...............81

IX. SUMMATION ON FIBER...............82

X. BONUS MATERIAL...............84
- Mother Dirt...............84
- GrainFields...............86

DIETARY FIBER BOOKS IN MY LIBRARY...............88
- Other Books That I Am Reading...............90

GLOSSARY...............92

ADDITIONAL REFERENCE MATERIAL...............103

# DISCLAIMER

This book is being presented to the reader for informational purposes only. It is meant to assist the general public in learning about dietary fiber and the microbiome. Nothing in this book is intended to serve as legal, medical, scientific, or spiritual advice in *any* matter; it is for educational purposes *only*. Each reader will and must draw their own unique conclusions about the material presented, and if the reader attempts to implement said material, that is entirely their responsibility.

The information provided in this book is designed to provide helpful information on the subjects discussed. It is *not* meant to be used, nor *should* it be used, to diagnose or treat any medical condition; this is the sole purview of your physician. The publisher and author are *not* responsible for any specific health or allergic conditions that may require medical supervision and are not liable for any damages or negative consequences from any treatment, action, application, or preparation to any person reading or following the information in this book. References are provided for informational purposes only and do *not* constitute endorsement of any websites or other sources. Readers should be aware that the websites listed in this book may change.

This book is not intended as a substitute for the medical advice of physicians. The reader should regularly consult a physician in matters relating to his/her health and, in particular, with respect to any symptoms that may require diagnosis or medical attention. If you think you may be suffering from any medical condition, you should seek immediate medical attention. You should never delay seeking medical advice, disregard medical advice, or discontinue medical treatment because of any information in this book.

Without prejudice to the generality of the foregoing paragraph, we do not represent, warrant, undertake or guarantee:

1. that the information in the book is correct, accurate, complete or non-misleading;
2. that the use of the guidance in the book will lead to any particular outcome or result; or
3. in particular, that by using the guidance in the book you will have any result whatsoever.

If a section of this disclaimer is determined by any court or other competent authority to be unlawful and/or unenforceable, the other sections of this disclaimer continue in effect. If any unlawful and/or unenforceable section would be lawful or enforceable if part of it were deleted, that part will be deemed to be deleted, and the rest of the section will continue in effect.

Nothing in this paper should be considered medical advice. For the treatment of any medical condition, you must seek the advice of a trained, medical doctor. This paper is *not* written with any specific products in mind but, rather, as a research of what is currently known about dietary fiber in general regarding nutrition.

# ACKNOWLEDGEMENTS

This book is dedicated to my parents, Marie D. Radatti and Vincent J. Radatti, and to my Aunts and Uncles and friends. These people made me who I am. To the divine spirit who made all possible, including the miracle of life.

*Additional Thanks to My Patron Saints:* Saint Jude Thaddeus, Mother Mary, and Saint Rita

Appreciation to Barbara Lynn Higgins, faithful researcher, editor, proof-reader, and all-around kibbitzer.

The cover photograph was licensed from istockphoto.com.

Explicate permission to quote other authors are contained within the text. All trademarks are the trademarks of their respective owners.

Finally, this book is dedicated to you, my readers. May the knowledge contained herein help you to avoid some of the pain I have experienced due to it's inaccessibility.

## **COPYRIGHT NOTICE AND EDITIONS**

Copyright © June 2018 by Peter V. Radatti. All rights reserved.

All rights reserved under United States law and International law, including, but not limited to, the Berne Convention. This work is *not* in the public domain.

        ISBN-13:    978-1545015421
        ISBN-10:    1545015422

# PREFACE – PLEASE READ

I am not a medical doctor (MD), a scientist, or even involved in the health or biological industries. I am just someone with a thirst for knowledge who is willing to share his opinion based on what he has read. Hopefully, what I have read, and decided to accept as fact, is true. In all cases, you will have to judge what I have presented for your scrutiny and decide for yourself, with the help of trained medical doctors to determine if anything I wrote is of value to you.

# Origins

This book started as a white paper on dietary fiber, entitled "Should Dietary Fiber Be Considered an Essential Nutrient?" That paper was published in June of 2012. The second paper, "You Are Not A Human", was presented at a conference in October, 2016. The third paper, "You Have 3 Brains", was written between February and March of 2017, and all three documents, along with updates and new material, were then combined into this book.

I wrote this book because I couldn't find one like it. It is my hope that I have succeeded in writing a popular reader on the subject of dietary fiber that explains what is known, some of what is *not* known, and why anyone should care. I, sometimes, have to use technical wording, but my aim is for this book to be readable by the general public.

# The Microbiome

This book is about dietary fiber and, because of it's topic, it is also about the *microbiome* of the gut. The microbiome is the low hanging fruit in medical science. Many of the advances that will happen in the next few dozen years will come from study of this entity. Dietary fiber is the food that feeds the gut's microbiome and, as such, has a singular effect on health.

# The Role of the Physician

This book is not intended as a substitute for the medical advice of physicians. The reader should regularly consult a physician in matters relating to his/her health and, in particular, with respect to any symptoms that may require diagnosis or medical attention. If you think you may be suffering from any medical condition, you should seek immediate medical attention. You should never delay seeking medical advice, disregard medical advice, or discontinue medical treatment because of information in this book.

# Footnotes

If you decide to follow in my footsteps and do this research for yourself (which is both suggested and fascinating), you will need to read my footnotes and book references. Most of them are references as to where I originally got my information. There is also additional reference section in the back of the book.

Yes, there are a lot of footnotes. Why? It is because the research out there is so confusing and, oftentimes, self-contradictory. Most of it is early research, a little of it has already been dis-proven or is currently in question, and some really basic facts are not even fully understood. Industry, and the politicians, have also created considerable controversy for their own purposes or through lack of knowledge. For this reason, and also to provide reference to *real* medical professionals, I footnote liberally. This is because I myself read footnotes. I believe them to be important and makes understanding the content of the book easier.

## **Conspiracy Theories**

If you do this research on your own, you will start to run into some conspiracy writing; people expressing the opinion that our modern diet is designed to kill us off in order to avoid paying pensions, Social Security, or the costs of an aging public on government. I don't believe in this conspiracy at all. Why attribute to planning and effort what can easily be explained by greed and unscrupulous behavior? The theory of Occam's Razor makes me believe that the lessor evils of corruption and a lack of understanding are *far* more likely reasons than the planned genocide of entire generations. I also think that if elected officials actually understood the seriousness of what is happening, then greed would not sway their decisions. This is not to say that I believe all politicians are virtuous, but just that most are not evil.

## **Diversity of Research Findings**

As you read this book and follow the reference material, you will start to find that there are a lot of diverse opinions on this subject. Many of these opinions are contradictory. There are a lot of reasons for that, one of which is that there are many thousands of different types of dietary fiber, many of which have different effects on the body. Specific things, such as fiber particle sizes or their various combinations at the time of ingestion, can have a great influence on the body.

There is not a lot of research in the field of dietary fiber, which is a true tragedy. This field of research, while small, is fast moving and productive, so a lot of even *recent* information is just plain wrong. There is the argument about what *is* and *is not* dietary fiber. The legal definition of dietary fiber is not even *close* to being realistic or biologically correct. Basically, I have had to decide which authorities I wanted to trust and which ones I felt were incorrect or out-of-date while writing this book. As in everything, there are some superstar researchers that I tend to believe more than researchers that I haven't heard of. In the interest of fairness, I will often refer to contradictory information in my footnotes and reference material. I have tried my best to pick out the good stuff and to make it easier to understand. This was not a simple task. In addition, as time progresses, new ideas and research will enlighten us even more. I believe that dietary fiber is very important and will become a ground-breaking area of research in the future.

## **A Wonder Food?**

I also want to post a warning here. Many people have a tendency to read a book like this and jump off the deep end, believing that the subject matter is a "cure" for what ails them and is some new "wonder drug/food". This would be a mistake. Dietary fiber is important, and I believe it is critical to health, but it is *not* a cure all! There is no such thing as a cure-all.

If dietary fiber has a large effect on the health of our population, which I believe is true, it is only because it has been missing in our modern diets. If we were still eating like our ancestors were, this book wouldn't have reason to exist.

Finally, this book has been professionally fact-checked and reviewed by both a professional copy-writer and several lay-persons prior to publication. I refuse to waste your time or mislead you in any way with this work. Having said that, thank you for reading my book!

Peter V. Radatti
June 2018

# **FAIR DISCLOSURE**

I own a business that manufactures foods based on high fiber formulas. Radatti Foods, LLC is a start-up that is starting manufacturing in 2018. It exists because former customers crowd sourced the funds necessary to bring the company back to life. (www.radattifoods.com). It was not something I expected or even wanted to do! My friends kept asking me to bring the products back and I kept telling them no. When they asked what I would need to bring the company back I replied "start up expenses". They found it! Surprised me. Next time, I won't answer.

I did not write this book to enhance the company or sell products. I wrote this book for the same reason that I started the company, which is that I am totally fascinated with the subject of dietary fiber, the microbiome, and how they interact to create us and sustain our health. This book was me, pulling information together that I learned from many sources, while attempting to generate an easy-to-understand explanation of how it all works. I have only partly succeeded, but this is my best attempt to date. This field of study is vast and only just starting. We haven't even reached the low hanging fruit yet.

In addition, it is my opinion that if the knowledge in this book were common within the medical community, that multiple people I loved would still be alive today.

Radatti Foods does not believe it is easy to change dietary habits that we develop over a lifetime. Unfortunately those habits have been formed by governmental interference and industry. We have gotten used to taking highly processed foods as normal and desirable. Radatti Foods believes that instead of changing people to desire beneficial foods we should change the desired foods to be beneficial high quality foods. We do this by blending multiple dietary fibers until we arrive at something that is acceptable and healthy. Apparently that is a unique approach.

You may notice that I don't mention any of my products in this book. Fair is fair. This is an educational and opinion document, not a sales pitch. I don't even soft pitch products that I manufacture here. If you want to know more you will have to visit the website and look for yourself. Be warned that Radatti Foods does not retail or wholesale and finding product may be hard. That will either self-correct or become even harder in the future as the company succeeds or fails.

Radatti Foods, LLC.
http:\\www.radattifoods.com

The sole distributor for Radatti Foods is:

The Essence of Life,
451 6th Avenue
Brooklyn, NY. 11215.
Phone: +1 (718) 788-8783.

# I: WHAT IS DIETARY FIBER?

From the 1800's thru to around 1960, every grandmother could easily answer the question, "What is dietary fiber?" Not that it was *called* dietary fiber; it was called *roughage*. Generally, it was understood to be the edible, but indigestible, parts of plants, such as the woody or structural sections of broccoli or celery. While people back then may not have known about all of the health reasons of eating fiber, they clearly understood some of the easier-to-observe benefits.

One of the historically-known benefits was that roughage helped prevent constipation and intestinal blockages, which could cause a painful death if not treated properly. Many Colonial American pharmaceutical books contained recipes for laxatives, partially due to a medical theory of the time concerning retained poisons in the gut. A review of the supplies of Lewis & Clark's 1806 expedition to explore and map the "west" included 50 dozen doses of a laxative called "Dr. Rush's patented Thunderclapper pills." Clearly, there were good reasons for eating healthy vegetables and fruits!

Today, constipation is still a common medical problem, although it tends to affect the institutionalized elderly and users of opioid pain killers the most. Lack of intestinal movement can require manual removal of waste matter in severe cases in order to avoid death or damage to the colon. Those were simpler times. Now, in our scientifically bright and shiny world, the answer to "what is dietary fiber" is no longer simple. Scientifically speaking, dietary fiber is a general class of chemicals called *polysaccharides*. In Latin, *poly* means "many", while *saccharides* means "sugar". This is not table sugar, but is made up of long chains of sugars that the human body is unable to digest. These polysaccharides were then scientifically broken down into many sub-classes.

The *real* problem is that "dietary fiber" has become a marketing term. There is money to be made, and any time there is money to be made, there will be politicians. Any time you add politicians to the works, everything becomes confusing. Up becomes down, down becomes left and nothing is right. The term "dietary fiber" has become anything the government says it is, including things that clearly are *not* dietary fiber.

Here's what we actually know: dietary fiber comes in two forms; water-*soluble* and water-*insoluble*. The plant-based insoluble fibers that exist in nature are called cellulose, hemicellulose, or lignin. That is not, however, everything that can be *legally* be called insoluble dietary fiber.

Additional compounds legally considered to be fiber are *chitin* and *Resistant Starch*.

## Water-Insoluble Fibers

Lets take a quick look at the definition of these different types, starting with insoluble fibers that comprise a plant's structure:

>*Cellulose* – found in fruits, cereals, vegetables and all plant life.
>*Hemicelluose* – found in bran, legumes, cereals, and timber. This is further broken down into *hexose*, which is from barley and wheat, and *pentose*, from oats and rye.

*Lignin* – found in vegetables, cereals, beans, the stones of fruits, and lumber.

*Xanthan Gum* –This comes from the Zanthomonas bacteria that is contained in sugar substrate.

Now for the "political gift" to insoluble fiber:

*Chitin* – this is the exoskeleton from insects, crustaceans, and some fungi. Basically, the crunchy parts, like shells. Yes, this is edible, but even if you may not want to eat it, you already are. Chitin is used in some processed foods, especially where the chitin contains useful colors. Chitin is "natural", therefore it serves as one of the possible "all natural food colorings" you see on food packaging. It can even be harvested from organically-grown bugs. I would be very surprised if anyone has studied the effects of chitin on human health. My guess is that it does not have the benefits of real dietary fiber, but it probably has no detrimental effects beyond "the yuck factor". People have been eating bugs, fungi, and crustaceans, such as shrimp and, therefore, chitin, forever. In fact, it is a staple in many third-world countries.

*Resistant Starch* – There are many types of resistant starch. They are generally categorized as one of three types: R1, R2, or R3. The R1 starch is usually found in the protective coating on fruit and nut shells, and some seeds. The R2 starch is similar, but is considered granular, while the R3 starch is called a retrograded starch. Resistant starch is most often extracted from legumes, high amylose corn, bananas, high amylose wheat, barley, etc…

My problem with calling resistant starch "dietary fiber" is that it is a *starch,* not a fiber. It is *resistant* to digestion but is not *indigestible*. In other words, this product *can* be put in our foods and called "dietary fiber" but it is not known if it contains any of the *benefits* of dietary fiber. Yes, it is food. No, it shouldn't hurt you. No, it is not really dietary fiber. On the other hand, Resistant Starch may be good for you in ways similar to fiber. Resistant Starch has been used to improve nutrition, blood sugar management, insulin insensitivity[1] [2] [3], irregularities[4], diarrhea[5] [6] [7] and to alleviate the symptoms of ulcerative colitis.[8] These same benefits exist in dietary fiber, so why bother with resistant starch? Answer: It costs less.

---

[1] Robertson, M. Denise; Wright JW; Loizon E; Debard C; Vidal H; Shojaee-Moradie F; Russell-Jones D; Umpleby AM (28 June 2012). "Insulin-sensitizing Effects On Muscle And Adipose Tissue After Dietary Fiber Intake In Men And Women With Metabolic Syndrome". Journal of Clinical Endocrinology & Meta-bolism. 97 (9):3326–32. doi:10.1210/jc.2012-1513. PMID 2274 5235.

[2] Kevin, Maki; Pelkman CL; Finocchiaro ET; Kelley KM; Lawless AL; Schild AL; Rains TM (April 2012). "Resistant Starch From High-Amylose Maize Increases Insulin Sensitivity In Overweight And Obese Me". journal of Nutrition. 142 (4): 717–23. doi:10.3945/jn.111.152975.PMC 3301990. PMID 2235 7745.

[3] Johnston, KL; Thomas EL; Bell JD; Frost GS; Robertson MD (April 2010). "Resistant Starch Improves Insulin Sensitivity In Metabolic Syn-Drome". Diabetic Medicine. 27 (4): 391–397. doi:10.1111/j.1464-5491.2010. 02923.x. PMID 20536509.

[4] Phillips, Jodi; Muir JG; Birkett A; Lu ZX; Jones GP; O'Dea K (July 1995). "Effect Of Resistant Starch On Fecal Bulk And Fermentation-Dependent Events In Humans". American Journal of Clinical Nutrition. 62 (1): 121–130.

[5] Ramakrishna, BS; Venkataraman S; Srinivasan P; Dash P; Young GP; Binder HJ (February 2000). "Amylase-resistant Starch Plus Oral Rehydration Solution For Cholera". The New England Journal of Medicine. 342: 308–313. doi:10.

# Water-Soluble Fiber

There are thousands of water soluble fibers and we are lucky to have them. Wonderful foods like apple pie, jellies and jams wouldn't exist without them.

Water soluble dietary fibers have traditionally been called gums. This separates them from other forms of gels, such as protein-based gelatins. <u>Gelatins are meat-, fish-, or foul-based.</u> It is the gel that develops when you refrigerate cooked meat. This is most commonly used in fruit gelatin (think Jello® brand gelatin) and in gummy candies.

---

1056/ NEJM 200002033420502. PMID 10655529.

[6] Raghupathy, P; Ramakrishna BS; Oommen SP; Ahmed MS; Priyaa G; Dziura J; Young GP; Binder HJ (2006). "Amylase-resistant Starch As Adjunct To Oral Rehydration Therapy In Children With Diarrhea". Journal of Pediatric Gastroenterology and Nutrition. 42 (4):362–368. doi:10.1097/01.mpg.0000214163. 83316. 41. PMID 16641573.

[7] Ramakrishna, Balakrishnan S.; Subramanian V; Mohan V; Sebastian BK; Young GP; Farthing MJ; Binder HJ (2008). "A Randomized Controlled Trial Of Glucose Versus Amylase Resistant Starch Hypo-Osmolar Oral Rehydration Solution For Adult Acute Dehydrating Diarrhea". PLoS ONE. 3 (2): e1587. Doi:10.1371/journal.pone.0001587. PMC 2217593. PMID 18270575.

[8] James, S. "P208. Abnormal Fibre Utilisation And Gut Transit In Ulcerative Colitis In Remission: A Potential New Target For Dietary Intervention". presen-tation at European Crohn's & Colitis Organization meeting, Feb 16-18, 2012 in Barcelona, Spain. European Crohn's & Colitis Organization. Retrieved 25 September 2016.

When you make natural fruit preserves, jams, or even pie fillings from fruit, you will notice that, after boiling for a sufficient period of time, the liquid gels after cooling. Basically, natural jellies and jams are gums. Chewing gum, though, is not really gum. Or, at least, not any more.

A few of the more common types of water soluble dietary fibers are fructans, polyuronides, monosaccharides, and raffinoses. There are also many artificial gums, such as lactulose, which exist in synthetic disaccharides and polydextrose, which is derived from synthetic polymers. A polymer is a chain of repeating sub-units bound together in various forms, short or long, such as plastics and resins.

> *Fructans* – the most famous version of a fructan is *Inulin*. It is often found in chicory, topinambour (Jerusalem artichoke), agave, asparagus, leeks, garlic, onions, yacon, jicama, and wheat, among other plants. Chemically, fructans are a polymer of the fructose sugar. Short-chained fructans are called fructo-oligosaccharides. You will commonly see this listed as an ingredient.
>
> *Polyuronides* – There are several different types of this fiber. The most famous is *pectin*. Apple pectin is often used in fruit jellies, jams, pie fillings, and more foods than I care to name. Completely natural and delicious! The Merriam-Webster dictionary defines polyuronide as "a polymeric substance consisting of uronic acid units with glycosidic linkages, often in combination with monosacchrides and occurring widely in plants (as in gums and pectic substances) and in soil." This means that it is a long chain, natural chemical made of uronic acid and sugars.

Polyuronides may actually be the super star of gum fibers; inexpensive, natural, and containing multiple substances which may be beneficial to health. Don't forget that they also make a great pie!

### Soluble vs. Insoluble: Benefits[9]

| SOLUBLE | INSOLUBLE |
|---|---|
| Prolongs stomach emptying so sugar is absorbed slower | Promotes regular bowel movement |
| Binds with fatty acids | Prevents constipation |
| Lower total cholesterol & LDL | Removes toxins quickly |
| Regulates blood sugar for people with diabetes | Maintains optimal balance of good microbes |
| Reduces risk of heart disease | May help prevent cancer |

## II. DEFINING DIETARY FIBER

Let's get back to the definition of what a dietary fiber is by looking at how other organizations define it.

According to the *IOM (The Institute of Medicine*[10]), dietary fiber is a combination of lignin and non-digestible carbohydrates that are naturally found in plants. These functional fibers are particularly non-digestible carbohydrates that have the tendency to be advantageous in

---

[9] https://www.uccs.edu/Documents/healthcircle/pnc/health-topics/ Soluble_ Insoluble_Fiber.pdf

[10] Institute of Medicine; Food and Nutrition Board. Dietary Reference Intakes: Energy, Carbohydrates, Fiber, Fat, Fatty Acids, Cholesterol, Protein And Amino Acids. Washington DC: National Academies Press; 2005.

the human body. Based on this, total fiber is the combination of both dietary and functional fibers.

My objection here is to the words "functional fiber". As far as I am concerned, there is no such thing. Either something is dietary fiber, or it is not. For example, a bicycle is not a functional automobile, even though it has some similar features.

Now lets see what the *politicians* have to say on the subject.

*The Codex Alimentarius Commission*[11] infers that dietary fibers are those carbohydrates polymers that possess over ten monomeric (same named) units and are not broken down by the effects of the endogenous (internally-secreted) enzymes contained in the small intestine of the human body.

Technically this is correct. It is *not* all-encompassing, but for what it does cover, it is correct. This definition adds nothing new, defines *something* but not the *entire* thing, is technically correct AND technically incorrect at the same time, and leaves everyone who reads it either confused or unsatisfied.

The next authority is much more to my liking, as far as accuracy goes.

---

[11] Codes Alimentarius Commission; Food and Agriculture Organization; World Health Organization. Report Of The 30th Session Of The Codex Committee On Nutrition And Foods For Special Dietary Uses. ALINORM 9/32/26.2009 [CITED2012March27].www.codexalimentarius.net/downlo ad/report/710/ al32_26e,pdf

*The American Association of Cereal Chemists*[12] has a very different view on the definition. They refer to dietary fiber as:

> "the analogous carbohydrate, which is that edible portion of plants which resists the digestion and absorption functions in the small intestines of human beings, as well as having partial or complete fermentation in the large intestine."

Dietary fiber, according to them, includes oligosaccharides, lignin, polysaccharides, and other plant substances. They aid in promoting favorable conditions in the body, such as the attenuation of blood cholesterol, regulation of bowel function, and blood sugar management.

Due to all of these confusing definitions, there are a lot of chemicals which are called dietary fiber which probably shouldn't be. In fact, the most common use of these chemicals is in children's packaged, cold breakfast cereals. Dietary fibers, especially gums, are extremely useful to the food processing industry. For that reason, they are often extracted from natural plants and refined, which I find acceptable. The fiber is not really changed in any way and can be added to foods to enhance their properties. Examples of such foods are shakes, frozen foods, ice cream, and traditionally-made fruit pies.

**My simple definition of fiber is *"the edible, but indigestible, parts of plants".***

---

[12] American Association of Cereal Chemists. The Definition Of Dietary Fiber: Report Of The Dietary Fiber Definition Committee To The Board Of Directors Of The American Association Of Cereal Chemists. Cereal Foods World. 2001; 46:112-26.

As you can see, lots of stuff called fiber fails that simple definition. Of course, there are also a lot of things that *do* fit that definition that you really shouldn't eat, but we'll leave that to another day.

# **Understanding the Role of Dietary Fiber**

Dietary fiber is not well understood. There is a lot of wrong information in the public about dietary fiber, but there are also many anecdotal studies indicating that, where a traditional diet of high fiber and natural foods are replaced with a modern diet of low fiber and processed foods, health deteriorates. Some studies indicate fiber may reduce the risk of heart disease, type 2 diabetes, high blood pressure, and breast and colon cancers.[13] It can help you lose weight by replacing high-calorie, high-carbohydrate foods with no-calorie, no-carbohydrate fiber. It may also help block the gut's absorption of calories while providing indirect biochemical benefits to the human body, regulating the digestion process, and promoting a sense of fullness after eating.

As was said before, all dietary fiber is from plant sources and is broken into two main categories; water-soluble and water-insoluble. Water-soluble fibers are also called gums. All plants contain both types of fiber in various degrees. The *insoluble* fibers are generally the structural parts of the plant, like stems or roots, while the soluble fibers are generally the water-filled parts of the plant, like leaves or fruit. Since the soluble fibers carry so much water, eating them slows down the emptying of the stomach, making you feel fuller longer. Soluble fibers can also help lower LDL

---
[13] Prevention, Fiber Up Slim Down Cookbook by Rodale, Page VII

(so-called bad) cholesterol by decreasing its absorption.[14] Insoluble fiber is considered gut-healthy fiber because it allows for easier fecal management by the body, and is also digested by bacterial in the gut which produces important byproducts used by the body, such as enzymes.[15]

Insoluble fiber is actually the majority of fiber we eat when eating raw or cooked, natural fruits, nuts, and vegetables. This fiber, while technically insoluble, *can* hold water; it simply can't be broken down by the body for food. A traditional, whole foods diet, consisting mostly of vegetables, nuts, and fruits, is rich in both soluble and insoluble fiber.

## **What Does It Do?**

One of the reasons that fiber doesn't get the respect that it should is because it is not well-understood. Many professionals think that fiber enters and exits the body without chemical alteration. That is far from the truth. In fact the effects of fiber on the body are profound. Dietary fiber should be considered an essential nutrient, as critical to good health as Vitamin C.

Let's entertain the supposition that fiber enters and exits the body mostly unchanged, which we have already determined to be false. First off, fiber is digested by bacteria in the human gut. The amount of digestion is determined by many factors, including the health of the subject, the diversity of the bacteria, and the type of fiber. For

---

[14] WebMD http://www.webmd.com/diet/fiber-health-benefits-11/ insoluble-soluble-fiber

[15] Anderson JW, Baird P, Davis RH, et al. (2009). "Health Benefits Of Dietary Fiber". Nutr Rev. 67(4): 188-205. doi: 10.1111/ j.173-4887. 2009. 00189.x. PMID 19335713

example, in a mixed diet fed to healthy individuals, 70 to 80% of the fiber is digested during passage through the gut.[16] Cellulose fibers survive digestion better than water-soluble fibers. The significant fact here is that dietary fiber is, indeed, utilized by the body and is *not* expelled in its totality. In healthy individuals, only 17% of the solid matter in feces is fiber. An additional 55% is actually bacteria, undigested food, water, mineral salts, and dead cells.[17]

The liver generates a substance called *bile* to aid in the digestion of fats in the small intestine. Bile is made from cholesterol, which is why anything that increases the production of bile decreases bloodstream cholesterol. The body generally mistakes soluble fiber for fats for the purpose of bile generation; however, since fiber is not a fat, it is not digested by the bile. Bile is fat-soluble, so it binds up fat-soluble toxins in the intestines. Unfortunately, instead of the bile being expelled, it is reabsorbed back into the blood. This changes when in the presence of insoluble fiber. The bile salts and its load of toxins bind to the insoluble fiber which is then expelled from the body.[18] This provides a triple benefit to the body. It lowers cholesterol by a natural process, it gently sponges toxins and expels them from the intestines, and it acts as a stimulant for the liver and digestive processes. Increasing the production of bile may help to prevent the formation of bile stones in the gall bladder and bile ducts.

---

[16] Cummings, John H, The Effect Of Dietary Fiber On Fecal Weight And Compositio,n 0-8493-2387-8/01 (CRC 185)
[17] Dr. David Williams, Alternatives, May 2012, page 3 (J Med Microbiol 80; 13(1):45-56)(FASEB J 91;5(13):2856-2859)
[18] Dr. David Williams, Alternatives May 2012, Page 5

# The Bacteria Connection

Humans exist as a mix of human and other living organisms which normally live together in healthful, harmonious way.[19] Many of these organisms are bacteria, along with a few helpful fungi. Even some of what were once considered to be "harmful" bacteria are now thought to provide important benefits to humans when existing in balance.[20] These beneficial microorganisms are called *symbiotes*. Exactly what symbiotes are needed to promote human health is unknown and largely unstudied.

Bacteria digest the fiber in the gut. One of the results of this is the release of *Inositol* from the phytic acid found in insoluble fiber. Inositol improves the metabolism of cholesterol and helps manage depression, insomnia, and fibromyalgia. In addition, these same bacteria create Vitamin K, which helps the body manage bleeding and blood clotting; Biotin (B7); and Vitamin K2. The K vitamins help manage calcium levels in the blood and prevents the buildup of calcium in soft tissue. Since humans are unable to store much Vitamin K, a diet rich in both types of fiber is required, as these bacteria would otherwise have no food and produce no beneficial results for the body.

This paragraph is quoted from Wikipedia:

> "When soluble fiber is fermented in the gut, short-chain fatty acids (SCFA) are produced. SCFAs are involved in numerous physiological processes

---

[19] http://en.wikipedia.org/wiki/Symbiosis
[20] Dr. David Williams Alternatives May 2012, page 2. In addition see recent studies of Helicobacter pylori in Science News October 9, 1999. http://www.sciencenews.org/sn_arc99/ 10_9_99/bob1.htm

promoting health. Some of these may be to help stabilize blood glucose levels by acting on pancreatic insulin release and liver control of glycogen breakdown, stimulate gene expression of glucose transporters in the intestinal mucosa, regulating glucose absorption, provide nourishment of colonocytes, particularly by the SCFA butyrate, suppress cholesterol synthesis by the liver and reduce blood levels of LDL cholesterol and triglycerides responsible for atherosclerosis, lower colonic pH (i.e., raises the acidity level in the colon) which protects the lining from formation of colonic polyps and increases absorption of dietary minerals stimulate production of T helper cells, antibodies, leukocytes, cytokines, and lymph mechanisms having crucial roles in immune protection, improve barrier properties of the colonic mucosal layer, inhibiting inflammatory and adhesion irritants contributing to immune functions. SCFAs that are absorbed by the colonic mucosa pass through the colonic wall into the portal circulation (supplying the liver), and the liver transports them into the general circulatory system. Overall, SCFAs affect major regulatory systems, such as blood glucose and lipid levels, the colonic environment, and intestinal immune functions. The major SCFAs in humans are butyrate, propionate, and acetate, where butyrate is the major energy source for colonocytes, propionate is destined for uptake by the liver, and acetate enters the peripheral circulation to be metabolized by peripheral tissues."

# How Much Is Enough?

The University of Kentucky recommended in a paper that the dietary fiber intakes for children and adults should be 14 g/1000 kcal and point out that more research is needed. While this is a useful figure for industrial food designers it is not very useful for someone attempting to eat a fiber rich diet from their refrigerator.

A more useful figure is provided by the United States National Academy of Sciences, Institute of Medicine, which suggest that adults should consume 20–35 grams of dietary fiber per day, but the average American's daily intake of dietary fiber is only 12–18 grams.[21]

The American Dietary Association recommends a minimum of 20–35 g/day for a healthy adult, depending on calorie intake (e.g., a 2000 Cal/8400 KJ[22] diet should include 25 g of fiber per day). The ADA's recommendation for children is that intake should equal age in years plus 5 g/day (e.g., a 4 year old should consume 9 g/day). No guidelines have yet been established for the elderly or very ill.

The British Nutrition Foundation has recommended a minimum fiber intake of 18 g/day for healthy adults.

---

[21] Linus Pauling Institute at Oregon State University, http://en.wikipedia.org/wiki/Dietary_fiber

[22] Kilojoules. 1 kJ = 0.2 Calories (Cals); 1 Calorie = 4.2 kJs.

# Suggested Dietary Fiber in Grams Per Day (g/d)

| Sex Age | Mayo Clinic <50 | 50+ | British | ADA | Nat. Acad. of Sci. |
|---|---|---|---|---|---|
| Men | 38 g/d | 30 g/d | 18 g/d | 20-35 g/d | 20-35 g/d |
| Women | 25 g/d | 21 g/d | 18 g/d | 20-35 g/d | 20-35 g/d |

These figures are the suggested minimum values of grams per day of dietary fiber someone should eat to obtain benefits. Will there be more benefits with more fiber? Will eating too much fiber cause harm to the body? There is very little information to answer these questions and, therefore, they are unanswered. It is safe to say that eating more will not be harmful as long as it is kept within reasonable limits and is used in an acceptable form. It appears that the minimum amount of fiber to gain health benefits is somewhere between 18 and 38 grams of dietary fiber per day for healthy adults. For the sake of argument, let's call 35 grams per day for adults as the minimum daily intake of dietary fiber needed to provide benefits.

How much food do you have to eat to consume 35 grams per day of fiber? The Mayo Clinic has a guide to answer this question at http://www.mayoclinic.com/health/high-fiber-foods/NU00582. An extract of some of the more common foods are:

# Quantity of Food Needed to Obtain 35 Grams/Day of Dietary Fiber

| **Mayo Clinic Supplied Value** | **35 gms /day** |
|---|---|
| Raspberries 1 cup (8.0 gms) | 4.4 cups |
| Apple w/ skin 1 med. (5.5 gms) | 6.36 apples |
| Orange 1 medium (3.1 gms) | 11.29 oranges |
| Rye Bread 1 slice (1.9 gms) | 18.42 slices |
| Brown Rice, cooked (3.5 gms/cup) | 10 cups |
| Split peas, cooked, 1 cup (16.3 gms) | 2.14 cups |
| Boiled Broccoli 1 cup (5.1 gms) | 6.86 cups |

Clearly, *no* one will be willing to eat this much food, so alternatives must be found.

# The "Up" Side of Fiber

The University of Kentucky published a paper on the health benefits of dietary fiber[23]. Among these benefits, they found that people with a diet high in dietary fiber may be at significantly lower risk for developing coronary heart disease, stroke, hypertension, diabetes, obesity, and some gastrointestinal diseases. Increasing dietary fiber lowered blood pressure and serum cholesterol levels, significantly increased weight loss in obese individuals, and benefited the gastrointestinal disorders of gastroesophageal reflux disease, duodenal ulcer, diverticulitis, constipation, and hemorrhoids. They also found that increasing fiber in the diet improves hyperglycemia and insulin sensitivity in non-diabetic and diabetic individuals. Their paper points out that prebiotic dietary fiber may enhance immune function and that the benefits of fiber may be similar for both children and adults.

Since fiber appears to hold significant value for health, it stands to reason that it should increase life expectancy. There is, in fact, a study completed by the US National Institute of Health and the American Association of Retired People (NIH-AARP) that states,

> "We found that dietary fiber intake was significantly inversely associated with risk of total death in both men and women."[24]

---

[23] Anderson JW, Baird P, Davis RH Jr, Ferreri S, Knudtson M, Koraym A, Waters V, Williams CL, .Health Benefits Of Dietary Fiber. Source Department of Internal Medicine and Nutritional Sciences Program, University of Kentucky, Lexington, Kentucky. PMID: 19335713 [PubMed - indexed for MEDLINE]

[24] Yikyung Park, ScD; Amy F. Subar, PhD; Albert Hollenbeck, PhD; Arthur Schatzkin, MD, Dietary Fiber

This means that eating more fiber may *increase* your life expectancy!

Now, lets take a look at a quote from an *unrelated* book that has a chapter on fiber. The book is discussing refined foods vs. natural, unrefined foods.

> "The claim is largely the fact that the diets of people living in rural areas of Africa consist largely of fiber-rich unrefined cereals, and it is in these areas that coronary thrombosis and other diseases of affluence are rare."[25]

Cereals are *not* a natural part of the human diet, as cereals such as wheat and rice only entered the human diet less than 10,000 years ago[26], an extremely short period of time, when one considers all of human evolution. I disagree with Dr. Yudkin, who believes that sugar is more harmful than a lack of dietary fiber. Humans have been eating the only concentrated form of sugar, honey, that exists naturally in nature, since the evolution of the bee. It is my belief that concentrated sugar(s), in large quantities, can be very harmful to the human body and its biome, but that, to a certain extent, it is the lack of sufficient dietary fiber in the diet that exacerbates the negative effects of sugar.

---

Intake and Mortality in the NIH-AARP Diet and Health Study, Arch Intern Med. 2011;171(12):1061-1068.doi:10.1001/archinternmed.2011.18
http://archinte.jamanetwork.com/article.aspx?articleid=227566

[25] Pure, White, and Deadly, John Yudkin ISBN 978-0-14-312518-1, page 33

[26] Pure, White, and Deadly, John Yudkin, page 34

# The "Down" Side of Fiber

So, fiber is great, right? Is there *anything* wrong with dietary fiber? Unfortunately, there is no such thing as a free lunch. Everything has a benefit trade-off and dietary fiber is no exception. Dietary fiber may slow down the transit time of prescription drugs, causing unexpected serum levels of the drug in the bloodstream. This has been observed with opioids but is easy to manage by a trained medical professional.[27] In addition, mixing dietary fiber with opioids drugs may cause severe constipation or even an obstruction requiring medical intervention. Fiber may also bind to and expel some vital minerals, which could be a problem for people with nutritional deficiencies, but these are rare in developed nations. Finally, there is always the embarrassment of flatulence which is always present when bacteria are active in the gut. Since dietary fiber is food for the good bacteria, there may be increased flatulence; however, some people report a reduction in the amount of flatulence (passing gas) with continued use of dietary fiber.

There is also the evil twin of *good* dietary fiber, and that is *bad* dietary fiber. This substance is rare, natural, and insoluble. Sawdust is one example. It was, at one time, used as a filler in sausage, according to Upton Sinclair's book, "The Jungle"[77] [28]. Large-sized particles of such a fiber can block the movement of food through the intestinal tract and affect how quickly pathogenic bacteria can multiply in the gut, due to lack of bowel motility ushering it out. Such overgrowth can cause infections or inflammation within the intestinal wall, a condition which is known as

---
[27] An MD will know how much time delay is needed between ingestion of drugs and dietary fiber, if any.
[28] https://en.wikipedia.org/wiki/Sawdust

contrabiotic.[29] [30] It is a poorly-understood process which will not be explored at length in this book. Basically, don't eat rough-ground sawdust in your food for its cellulose!

Recently, the food industry has started to call some substances that would have never been called dietary fiber before, "functional" fiber[31], such as man-made chemicals and the products of bacteria and yeasts. In addition, the US Food and Drug Administration decided, in 2007, that the chemical *polydextrose* could legally be called fiber. This chemical is already in use in children's foods. The problem is that no one knows if these artificial dietary fibers have any of the helpful properties of *natural* fiber while legally being called fiber.[32]

One other consideration is that not all soluble fibers have the same effect on the human body. For example, Inulin, from chicory root, is considered a prebiotic, which promotes the growth of symbiotic (good) bacteria but doesn't lower cholesterol. These problems can be resolved by using a blend of many different dietary fibers which would then provide a wider spectrum of fiber-related benefits.

---

[29] Simpson, H; Campbell, BJ (2015). "Review Article. Dietary Fibre-Microbiota Interactions.". Aliment Pharmacol Ther. 42(2): 158-79. doi:10.1111/apt.13248. PMID 26011307.

[30] Simpson, H; Campbell, BJ; Rhodes, JM (2014). "IBD: Microbiota Manipulation Through Diet And Modified Bacteria.". Dig Dis. 32Suppl1: 13-25. doi:10.1159/000367821

[31] Rodale, Men's Health, November 2009 Page 102

[32] Rodale, Men's Health, November 2009 Page 104

**WARNING:** *Never* eat dry dietary fiber. That means Chia seeds, powered dietary fiber supplements, or any other dry fiber, including fiber-based products that are suppose to help you treat constipation. Doing so will earn you a quick trip to the emergency room at your local hospital. First off, *most* fibers will absorb many times their weight in water. For example, Chia seeds absorb *twenty-seven times* their weight in water. If you eat them dry, they absorb the water from your mouth and throat, which can cause you to choke to death. If it happens in your stomach, you could literally block your digestive track with the natural equivalent to concrete, *again* earning you a trip to the emergency room. To avoid all of these problems, **DO NOT EAT FIBER DRY!** It almost *never* exists in the dry form in nature, so you will never have that problem eating real food.

## **Synopsis**

Dietary fiber helps beneficial bacteria in the gut by providing their preferred food source, enabling them to grow rapidly and crowd out bad bacteria. These good bacteria also provide many biochemical benefits to the entire body, in addition to enhancing the immune system and synthesizing necessary hormones. Other fiber-related benefits that are *not* related to beneficial bacterial include: blood sugar moderation, increased movement of fecal matter through the gut which allows for easier bowel movements, and the gentle scrubbing of the intestinal walls that assists in the removal of non-beneficial bacteria, toxins, and parasites. It also assists the liver by removing bile salts, bearing excess cholesterol, from the gut.

While natural whole plant foods are the preferred form of dietary fiber, many believe that dietary fiber extracts from plant foods which are purified and concentrated are beneficial in aiding cases of abdominal discomfort, diarrhea and some forms of irritable bowel syndrome[33] [34], which cannot tolerate the actual fiber itself without distress. Some dietary fibers, such as inulin, are considered prebiotic and can help manage some inflammatory diseases of the bowel.[35]

Inulin is a very interesting dietary fiber, since it has properties that most fibers do not have, as well as effects on the human body that are very desirable. This does not, however, mean that it is the best or only fiber like it. It has some significant advantages, in that it is inexpensive and easy to extract from both Jerusalem artichokes and chicory roots, where it is abundant. Inulin is already used in many food products safely[36]. It is often used as a substitute for, or to enhance sweetness of, flour and/or fats. Inulin is both a digestable carbohydrate, in that a portion of it is digested

---

[33] Friedman G (September 1989). "Nutritional Therapy Of Irritable Bowel Syndrome". Gastroenteroly Clin North Am. 18 (3): 513–24. PMID 2553606.

[34] MacDermott RP (January 2007). "Treatment Of Irritable Bowel Syndrome In Outpatients With Inflammatory Bowel Disease Using A Food And Beverage Intolerance, Food And Beverage Avoidance Diet". Inflamm Bowel Dis. 13 (1): 91–6. doi:10.1002/ibd.20048. PMID 17206644.

[35] Ewaschuk JB, Dieleman LA (October 2006). "Probiotics And Pre-Biotics In Chronic Inflammatory Bowel Diseases". World J Gastro-enterol. 12 (37): 5941–50. PMID 17009391. Archived from the original on 13 September 2008.

[36] Kaur N, Gupta AK (December 2002). "Applications Of Inulin And Oligo-Fructose In Health And Nutrition" (Pdf). J Biosci. 27 (7): 703–14. doi:10.1007/BF02708379. PMID 12571376.

for energy while the remainder is fermented in the gut like a fiber, and a fructan dietary fiber. It is also considered a prebiotic, fermentable fiber.[37] As such, it can be used to reduce sugar content while providing a calorie savings of between 70% to 75%, while also being used to reduce fat content by providing a calorie savings of between 85% to 90%.

After digestion, inulin can enhance absorption of calcium[38], magnesium[39], and iron[40]. It is believed that this happens because of enhanced regulation of the genes which are responsible for transporting minerals through the membrane proteins in the colon wall. While it does all that, it is also believed to significantly increase the reproduction and well-being of various lactobacillus and bifidobacterium within the intestine. This is very desirable.

---

[37] Roberfroid MB (1 November 2007). "Inulin-type Fructans: Functional Food Ingredients". J Nutr. 137 (11 Suppl): 2493S–2502S. PMID 17951492.

[38] Abrams S, Griffin I, Hawthorne K, Liang L, Gunn S, Darlington G, Ellis K (2005). "A Combination Of Prebiotic Short- And Long-Chain Inulin-Type Fructans Enhances Calcium Absorption And Bone Mineralization In Young Adolescents". Am J Clin Nutr. 82 (2): 471–6. PMID 16087995.

[39] Coudray C, Demigné C, Rayssiguier Y (2003). "Effects Of Dietary Fibers On Magnesium Absorption In Animals And Humans". j Nutr. 133 (1): 1–4. PMID 12514257.

[40] Tako E, Glahn RP, Welch RM, Lei X, Yasuda K, Miller DD (2007). "Dietary Inulin Affects The Expression Of Intestinal Enter-Ocyte Iron Transporters, Receptors And Storage Protein And Alters The Microbiota In The Pig Intestine". Br J Nutr. 99 (Sep):1–9. doi:10.1017/S0007114507825128. PMID 17868492.

Inulin does have some significant problems, however. If it didn't, we would be eating it by the shovel-full. Inulin is not well tolerated, especially by people on certain types of drugs, as it can cause digestive difficulties, pain, and gassing issues.[41][42] This is not all bad news, though. Some clinical studies have indicated, on practical findings, that inulin can still be effective when taken at small dosages of 15-grams per day[43], minimizing digestive discomfort.

---

[41] Grabitske, Hollie A.; Slavin, Joanne L. (2009). "Gastro-intestinal Effects Of Low-Digestible Carbohydrates". Critical Reviews in Food Science and Nutri-tion. 49 (4): 327–360. doi: 10.1080/10408390802067126. PMID 19234944.

[42] Shepherd, Susan J.; Gibson, Peter R. (2006). "Fructose Mal-absorption and Symptoms of Irritable Bowel Syndrome: Guidelines for Effective Dietary Management". Journal of the American Dietetic Association. 106 (10): 1631–1639. doi:10. 1016/j.jada. 2006. \07.010. PMID 17000196.

[43] Liber, A.; Szajewska, H. (2013). "Effects Of Inulin-Type Fructans On Appetite, Energy Intake, And Body Weight In Children And Adults: Systematic Review Of Randomized Controlled Trials". Ann Nutr Metab. 63 (1–2):42–54.doi: 10.1159/0003 50312. PMID 23887189.

Some of the problems that specific dietary fibers have been shown to help is Crohn's disease[44], ulcerative colitis[45] [46] and Clostridium difficile.[47] Dietary fibers, which result in the production of specific short chain fatty acids, can lead to anti-inflammatory effects in the bowel.[48] [49] [50]

---

[44] Guarner F (April 2005). "Inulin And Oligofructose: Impact On Intestinal Diseases And Disorders". Br J Nutr. 93 Suppl 1: S61–5. Doi:10.1079/ BJN 20041345. PMID 15877897.

[45] Seidner DL, Lashner BA, Brzezinski A, et al. (April 2005). "An Oral Supplement Enriched With Fish Oil, Soluble Fiber, And Antioxidants For Corticosteroid Sparing In Ulcerative Colitis: A Randomized, Controlled Trial". Clin Gastroenterol Hepatol. 3 (4): 358–69. doi:10.1016/S1542-3565(04)00672-X. PMID 15822041.

[46] Rodríguez-Cabezas ME, Gálvez J, Camuesco D, et al. (October 2003). "Intestinal Anti-Inflammatory Activity Of Dietary Fiber (Plantago Ovata Seeds) In Hla-B27 Transgenic Rats". ClinNutr. 22 (5):463–71.doi:10.1016/S0261-5614(03) 00045-1. PMID 14512034.

[47] Ward PB, Young GP (1997). "Dynamics Of Clostridium Difficile Infection. Control Using Diet". Adv Exp Med Biol. 412: 63–75. PMID 9191992.

[48] Säemann MD, Böhmig GA, Zlabinger GJ (May 2002). "Short-chain Fatty Acids: Bacterial Mediators Of A Balanced Host-Microbial Relationship In The Human Gut". Wien Klin Wochenschr. 114 (8–9): 289–300. PMID 12212362.

[49] Cavaglieri CR, Nishiyama A, Fernandes LC, Curi R, Miles EA, Calder PC (August 2003). "Differential Effects Of Short-Chain Fatty Acids On Proliferation And

I personally believe that concentrated extracts of plant fibers, depending upon what they are, can be as or *more* useful to the human body than natural whole plant foods. One of the reasons for this is that it is a lot easier to eat a concentrated dietary fiber supplement than a whole mountain of food, which could cause its own kind of problem!

---

Production Of Pro- And Anti-Inflammatory Cytokines By Cultured Lymphocytes". Life Sciences. 73 (13): 1683–90. doi:10.1016/S0024-3205 (03)00490-9. PMID 12875900.
[50] Liber, A.; Szajewska, H. (2013). "Effects Of Inulin-Type Fructans On Appetite, Energy Intake, And Body Weight In Children And Adults: Systematic Review Of Randomized Con-trolled Trials". Ann Nutr Metab. 63 (1–2): 42–54. doi: 10.1159/ 0003 50312. PMID 23887189.

# III. THE EFFECT(S) OF DIETARY FIBER

Dietary fiber goes through the stomach and small intestines unbroken. Human digestion does not contain the enzymes and other chemicals used by herbivores to digest fiber. For this reason, fiber is passed mostly unchanged to the large intestine, where most of the effects take place.

Here's what we know so far (4 points):

> 1) Dietary fiber feeds the good bacteria in the microbiome.[51]
> 2) The microbiome has a large impact on the immune system and hormone-production system.
> 3) Dietary fiber and resistant starch reduce diabetic

---
[51] Simpson, H.L.; Campbell, B.J. (2015). "Review Article: Dietary Fibre-Microbiota Interactions". Alimentary Pharma-cology & Therapeutics. 42(2): 158-179. doi:10.1111/ apt.13248. PMID 26011307.

tendencies by an unknown, but well-observed, means.[52 53 54 55 56 57]

4) Fiber reduces bad cholesterol by means of bile salt absorption and excretion through the bowel.

In addition, there is some evidence that the effects of dietary fiber and high amylose-resistant starch may affect

---

[52] Weickert MO, Pfeiffer AF (2008). "Metabolic Effects Of Dietary Fiber Consumption And Prevention Of Diabetes". J Nutr. 138(3); 439-42. PMID 18287346

[53] Johnston, KL; Thomas EL; Bell JD; Frost GS; Robertson MD (2010), "Resistant Starch Improves Insulin Sensitivity In Metabolic Syndrome:" Diabetic Medicine.27(4):391-397.doi:10. 1111/j.1464-5491.2010.02923.x.PMID 20536509.

[54] Robertson, M. Denise; Currie JM; Morgan LM. Jewell DP; Frayn KN (2003). "Prior Short-Term Consumption Of Resistant Starch Enhances Postprandial Insulin Sensitivity In Healthy Subject" (PDF). Diabetologia. 46(5); 659-665. doi:10.1007/ s00125-003-1081-0. PMID 12712245.

[55] Robertson, M. Denise; Bickerton AS; Dennis AL; Vidal H; Frayn KN (2005). "Insulin-sensitizing Effects Of Dietary Resistant Starch And Effect On Skeletal Muscle And Adipose Tissue Metabolism". The American Journal of Clinical Nutrition. 82(3): 559-567. PMID 16155268.

[56] Maki, Kevin C.; Pelkman CL; Finocchiaro ET; Kelley KM; Lawless AL; Schild AL; Rains TM (April 2012)."Resistant Starch From High-Amylose Maize Increases Insulin Sensitivity In Overweight And Obese Men". Journal of Nutrition. 142(4): 717–723. doi:10.3945/jn.111. 152975. PMC 3301990. PMID 2235 7745.

[57] Robertson, M. Denise; Wright JW; Loizon E; Debard C; Vidal H; Shojaee-Moradie F; Russell-Jones D; Umpleby AM (28 June 2012). "Insulin-sensitizing Effects On Muscle

the triggering of genes, which can affect the function of the digestive system and the associated functions and flora. [58] This research is still in its early years.

## **You Are Not A Human!**

Would you consider early cars to be made from wood if less than 10% of the car was wood? No!

Early cars had wooden floors, seats, trim, dashboards and a few other parts, but cars were mostly metal; the most important parts, the engine and transmission, could *not* be made of wood. Most people would either consider the car to be made from metal or would, more correctly, identify the car as a composite of materials, with the exception of a handful of novelty cars whose chassis were made of wood.[59]

Using this logic, your body is not human! Only 10% of the cells that comprise your body are human. That is, 10% by cell count, not weight.

---

And Adipose Tissue After Dietary Fiber Intake In Men And Women With Metabolic Syndrome". Journal of Clinical Endocrinology & Metabolism. 97 (9): 3326–32. doi:10.1210/jc.2012-1513. PMID 22745235.

[58] Keenan, M.J.;Martin, R.J.; Raggio, A.M.; McCutcheon, K.L.; Brown, I.L.; Birkett, A.; Newman, S.S.; Skaf, J.; Hegsted, M.; Tulley, R.T.; Blair, E.;Zhou, J. (2012). "High-Amy-lose Resistant Starch Increases Hormones And Improves Structure And Function Of The Gastrointestinal Tract: A Microarray Study" Journal Of Nutrigenetics And Nutri-Genomics. 5(1): 26-44. doi: 10.1159/ 000335319. PMID 22516953.

[59] https://jalopnik.com/5870797/the-ten-coolest-wooden-cars-of-all-time/

Your body is 90% symbiotic bacteria and fungus. This bacteria is essential for life. Without it, you die.

Let me go further. Of the 10% of your body which is made up of human cells, where the DNA is considered "human", a *significant* part of the human cells are *not* human. The microchondria, for example, are the parts of your body that power the human cells, yet microchondria do not share *any* DNA with humans. The DNA in the microchondria is bacterial in nature.

**Defination of Mitochondria from Dictionary.Com**

**Mitochondrion**      *Plural,* **mitochondria**
> *"A structure in the cytoplasm of all cells except bacteria in which food molecules (sugars, fatty acids, and amino acids) are broken down in the presence of oxygen and converted to energy in the form of ATP[60]. Mitochondria have an inner and outer membrane. The inner membrane has many twists and folds (called cristae), which increase the surface area available to proteins and their associative reactions. The inner membrane encloses a liquid containing DNA, RNA, small ribosomes, and solutes. The DNA in mitochondria is genetically distinct from that in the cell nucleus, and mitochondria can manufacture some of their own proteins independent of the rest of the cell. Each cell can contain thousands of mitochondria, which move about producing ATP in response to the cell's need for chemical energy. It is thought that mitochondria originated as separate, single-celled organisms that became so symbiotic with their hosts*

---
[60] Adenosine Triphosphate. The fuel your cells run on. No ATP = No Life.

> *as to be indispensible. Mitochondrial DNA is thus considered a remnant of a past existence as a separate organism."*

Therefore, the part of your human cells that keeps them alive is bacterial in nature. To go further, many parts of the human DNA have been identified as having been supplied by bacterial and viral materials.

You now know that less than 10% of your body is "human" and, of the parts that *are* human, a critical part, the part that powers the human cells, is *not* human. Even the definition of human DNA includes DNA snips from other organisms.

This is not just true for humans. It is true for *all* living things, especially animals, but also plants.

What this means is that you are *not* fully human. Since that is the case, why do we ignore the non-human 90% of our bodies when discussing health?

# IV. SYMBIOTES!

Your bowels contain mostly symbiotic bacterial. They produce most of your immune system, many critical hormones, and digest significant parts of your food, and this is just the bacteria in your gut! The bacteria that is a significant part of your skin protect you from skin cancer, produces Vitamin D (a critical hormone), and provides much of what keeps your skin looking young and healthy.

Hippocrates declared, over 2000 years ago, that *"death sits in the bowels"*. This means that, when something goes wrong with these critical bacteria, then illness and death follow. What can go wrong? How about this, from the website entitled "Glyphosate Used With GMO Crops Under Attack for Disrupting Microbiome Science, or A Gut Feeling":

> "One species of *Clostridium* causes botulism and another causes a life-threatening condition the survival from which has been improving mostly because of the fecal transplant procedure. The study looked at the effects of glyphosate on these pathogenic bacteria and also on several important friendly bacterial strains. It turns out that the *Clostridium* and *Salmonella* are fairly resistant to glyphosate, while several friendly strands are moderately to highly susceptible to glyphosate, meaning that they might be killed off."[61]

---

[61]https://www.geneticliteracyproject.org/2014/12/05/glyphosate-used-with-gmo-crops-under-attack-for-disrupting-microbiome-science-or-a-gut-feeling/

What can cause the beneficial bacteria to die? It turns out that the number one cause of symbiotic death is a lack of dietary fiber in our diets. A strong second is the overuse of antibiotics in ourselves and in our food. A third is toxins. *glyphosate* (aka: Roundup) has been identified as a moderate toxin to good bacteria, while it has no effect on many forms of bad (pathogenic) bacteria.

We stress the beneficial bacteria that keeps us alive by not feeding them their preferred food, dietary fiber. We kill them with excessive antibiotics and we poison them with herbicides, fungicides, pesticides, artificial colors, sweeteners, and preservatives. We consume excessive amounts of sugar, which benefits the "bad" bacteria. Then we wonder how we could have set ourselves up for failure as a healthy person.

A new kind of treatment, fecal transplants, has been used to save lives in Europe and elsewhere. It is only just becoming available in the United States, primarily due to "the yuck factor" and regulatory delays. In addition to saving lives, it has been indicated as a medical treatment for obesity and many other problems, including some physiological ailments. Here is what Drexel Medicine Gastroenetrology says about Fecal Microbiota Transplant:

> Patients with C.Diff in their digestive tracts, usually from taking too many antibiotics, causes problems with diarrhea, abdominal pain, bloating, fatigue, and fever. In addition, Fecal Transplant may assist in Inflammatory Bowel Disease, Irritable Bowel Syndrome, Crohn's Disease, and Ulcerative Colitis. There are also suggestions that it can assist in non-digestive conditions, including neurological,

rheumatologic, and cardiovascular disease. You can view a list of ongoing studies at clinicaltrials.gov.[62]

The problem with this technique is that we are really stumbling in the dark. Modern science has no idea what most of the bacteria that sustains us is or how they interact with each other *or* us. In addition, it now appears that some bacteria may, in fact, cause long term illnesses years later. The source material must be very well screened and we are only just beginning to learn how.

Why not just culture the needed bacteria and use that instead of transplanted fecal matter? The reason is because there are thousands of different bacteria needed to keep us alive and we don't know what most of them are or do. We can *see* them, but we don't know what they *are*. In addition, fecal transplant, as practiced in Europe, is as safe as current science can allow.

## **Effects on Age, Sleep, and Circadian Rhythm**

In the last couple of decades, scientists have come to a new appreciation of the function of the microbiome of the gut. They now understand how these microbes, once grossly underestimated, can affect the healthy inner workings of our *entire* bodies, not just the gut:

> "We now recognize they're essential to our health, participating in many important physiological functions such as digestion and metabolism of foods, and immune responses and inflammation; disruption of the gut microbiota might then

---

[62] http://www.drexelmedicine.org/patient-services/gastro-enterology/services/ fecal-microbiota-transplant/

contribute to a variety of conditions including child-hood asthma, obesity, colitis and colon cancer."[63]

Researchers have discovered that the microbiome of the gut is different at different times of day. This is consistent with the body's circadian variations in other areas, such as metabolism, appetite, sleep, hormones, etc. In fact, not only do the microbes in the gut change their activity and output, with the time of day, they also can change location in the colon.

Changes in the time of feeding, a massive die-off of microbiota in the gut, or the introduction of poisons or toxins into the system, can affect how the liver, for example, functions, dependent upon the time of day. The body can handle such stresses better early in the morning, whereas it will suffer more from the ill effects of such issues in the evening. Such findings can influence things like the optimum times for taking medications, thereby minimizing side effects and improving effectiveness.

Gut microbes, it seems, work in a community rather than as individuals, so a change in the output of one species can influence them all. One species may need what another species of microbe produces at a given time of day. Plus, whether the microbes are being fed in the day or at night also makes a great deal of difference in microbe function.[64]

---

[63] Stevens, Richard G., "Circadian Rhythms And The Micro-biome: Disrupting Daily Routine Of Gut Microbes Can Be Bad News For The Whole Body", www.salon.com, December 24, 2016
[64] Ibid (same as above)

This can be seen clearly in the effect of the gut microbiome on obstructive sleep apnea. Scientists have found that this ailment occurs most often in people who are obese or diabetic. The presence of high amounts of fat in the gut changes the microbiome balance, a situation called *dysbiosis*. In one study, where thin subjects with pre-existing apnea were fed a high-fat diet, they did *not* become overweight, but they *did* become hypertensive. This showed that it was the *combination* of apnea and high-fat diet that caused the hypertension. Without the fatty diet, the subject with apnea continued to have normal blood pressure because of the normal gut microbiome.[65]

While the time of day and diet may affect the microbiome, age itself doesn't have to affect it. Studies in China have illustrated that, if a person is healthy *at any* age, their microbiomes will be very similar. As Greg Gloor, a professor at Western's Schulich School of Medicine & Dentistry, stated:

> "The main conclusion is that if you are ridiculously healthy and 90 years old, your gut microbiota is not that different from a healthy 30 year old in the same population….This demonstrates that maintaining diversity of your gut at your age is a biomarker of healthy aging, just like low cholesterol is a biomarker of a healthy circulatory system."[66]

---

[65] Baylor University, "Obstructive Sleep Apnea-Induced Hyper-tension Linked To Gut Microbiome", medicalxpress.com, February 9th, 2016

[66] Biomarker, Microbiome, "Gut Microbiota Of Healthy Elders Not Different From 30 Year-Olds, Study Shows," www.news-medical.net, October 11th, 2017

It might be possible to reset an elderly person's microbiome to that of a 30 year old by adding diverse microbes to the older person's system or, conversely, make a younger, less healthy person healthy again by making their microbiome more like a healthy senior's.

A healthy microbiome has an anti-aging affect on the body. Supplying *fiber* can have a multitude of effects by:

> 1) cutting cholesterol, for healthy heart and blood vessels,
> 2) preventing diabetes, by managing levels of sugar in the blood and gut,
> 3) controlling weight, and cutting down on all obseity-related diseases,
> 4) reducing inflammation, and all diseases related to it,
> 5) protecting joints, by reducing inflammation and weight-induced stress, and
> 6) boosting good bacteria in the gut, allowing it to function optimally to maintain health.[67]

## Microbiome Players

The following information is quoted from the book **"The Symbiont Factor, How the Gut Microbiome Redefines Health, Disease, and Humanity," by Richard Matthews.**[68] (Used with explicit permission of the author.) I recommend this book highly, as I quote from the 2014 edition, pages 348 to 354. This topic will be the most

---

[67] Wadyka, Sally, "The Surprising Anti-Aging Benefits of Fiber," www.consumerreports.org, February 15th, 2018

[68] Matthews, Richard, "The Symbiont Factor, How the Gut Microbiome Redefines Health, Disease and Humanity". ISBN-13: 978-150055944, ISBN-10: 1500553948.

important area of research for the next 100 years and, of the dozen or so books I have on the subject, this book is the best and most scientific. Here is a list of known symbionts:

**Streptococcus Thermophilus**
- Prevents bacterial translocation during laparoscopic surgery (Sahin)
- Helps pregnant women maintain insulin function, preventing gestational diabetes (Asemi)
- Fights Clostridum difficile infections (Kolling)

**Loctobacillus Plantarum**
- Lowers cholesterol (Oner)
- Protects against influenza virus (Park)
- Lowers BMI (body mass index) and blood pressure (Sharafedtinov)
- Reduces Immunoglobulin E anaphylactic allergic reactions (Yoshida)
- Protects NK (natural killer) immune cells from gamma radiation (Lee)

**Lactobacills Rhamnosus**
-Helps to prevent or treat MRSA (Methicilline Resistant Staphylococcus aureus) (Sikorska)
-Protects colon muscle from LPS-induced damage (Ammososcato)
-Prevents rhinovirus (colds) in premature infants (Luoto)
-Protects against cancer-causing effects of ultraviolet light (Weill)
-Protects intestines against damage from radiation (Ciorba)

**Lactobacillus Casei**
- Helps prevent breast cancer (Kaga, Toi), along with soy isoflavones in diet
- Restores damaged dendritic cell function in ulcerative colitis (Mann)

-Inhibits growth of liver cancer cells (Han)

**Lactobacillus Fermentum**

-Inhibits growth of bacteria that causes tooth decay (Chen, Elavarasu)

- Improves tight junctions between intestinal cells (preventing leaky gut) (Sultana)

- Protects liver cells from damage from extended alcohol exposure (Park). A type of kombucha, can be made by L.fermentum-fermenting green tea.

- Reduces the effects of metabolic syndrome/insulin resistance (rate model of human function) (Tomaro-Duchesneau)

**Bifidobacterium Infantis**

-Modulates inflammatory responses of the host (Groeger)

-Programs the immune system and reduces allergies (Toh)

**Bifidobacterium Breve**

- Protects skin against ultraviolet light damage (Sugimoto)

- Protects kidneys against formation of calcium oxalate stones (Giardina)

- Prevents airway constriction and asthma (Sagar), when combined with oligosaccharides (found in Jerusalem artichokes, asparagus, leeks and onions)[69]

**Bifidobacterium Bifidum**

- Lowers blood pressure (Gonzalez-Gonzalez)

- Reduces total cholesterol and LDL cholesterol (Bordoni)

- Helps prevent or treat Clostridium difficile infections (Sikorska)

---

[69] PVR-- the book says that oligosaccharides are a non-digestible fiber, but that is now known to not be true. It is legally dietary fiber, but it is digestible and, therefore, not an actual fiber.

### Lactobacillus Acidophilu

- Inhibits growth of Salmonella (Scapin)
- Reduces inflammation in intestinal epihelial cells (Borthakur)
- Modulates inflammatory gene expression in overweight patients (Zarrati)
- When given to the mother of low birth weight infants who were breastfed, it reduced the incidence of necrotizing enterocolitis, "death of intestine," which can be fatal (Benor)
- Reduces inflammation and oxidative stress in atherosclerosis (Chen)
- Protects intestinal epithelial cells in radiation exposure (Chitapanarux)

### Combinational Benefits

Some benefits have only been shown in combinations of several probiotic species:

1) Reducing inflammation and oxidative stress in Type 2 diabetics (Asemi, testing yogurt with cultures of Streptococcus thermophilus, Lactobacillus bulgaricus, Lactobacilus acidophilus LA5 and Bifidobacterium animalis BB12)
2) Reducing inflammation and muscle atrophy in leukemia (mouse model of leukemia, studied with Lactobacillus reuteri 100-23 and Lactobacillus gasseri 311476) (Bindels)
3) Reduced severity of myocardial infarction (heart attack) and improved recovery from it using Goodbelly®, a popular probiotic drink that contains Lactobacillus plantarum 299v (Lam)

4) Preventing, reducing spread of, and improving treatment of colorectal cancer using combinations of Lactobacillus and Bifidobacterium (Geier)

## **Food-Like Probiotic Supplements**

Some of the best probiotics (other than those available as probiotic capsule supplements) you can introduce into your body are more like foods or beverages. Here I will review some of the most common and most available ones. You may have been consuming some of these for years and not realized just how healthy they are!

### Kombucha: Benefits of a Probiotic Drink

Kombucha is estimated to have been fermented and consumed for the last 2000 years. One of the more common fermented drinks/foods that is not beer or wine, it is available in many grocery and health food stores, as well as being easy to make at home. There is a plethora of evidence for the health benefits of kombucha tea! One study concluded that kombucha can prevent or heal diabetes (Aloulou).

Different brands have their own bacterial profiles, and the home-brewed variety also has an assortment of beneficial bacteria and yeasts. Generally, home-brewed kombucha begins with a SCOBY, or Symbiotic Colony Of Bacteria and Yeast. These are the actual culture that ferments the sweet tea and forms kombucha.[70]

---

[70] PVR—The following bacilli are discussed in terms of being part of Kombucha. You will notice some of the properties have changed.

**Bacillus Coagulans**
- Helps to treat, prevent, or recover from Clostridum difficile infections (Fitzpatrick, 3 studies)
- Antimicrobial activity against pathogenic bacteria (Honda)
- Anti-inflammatory and immune-modulating (Jensen)
- Reduces amount of diarrhea with irritable bowel syndrome (Dolin)
- Reduces some of the symptoms of rheumatoid arthritis (RA) by immune system modulation (Mandel)
- Reduces excess gas production and pain/ discomfort (Kalman)
- Improves pain and bloating from IBS (Hun)
- Enhances T-cell response to respiratory viral infections (Baron)

**Lactobacillus Paracasei**
- Elimination or reduction of MRSA (Methicillin Resistant Staphylococcus Aureus) infection (Sikorska)
- Prevention of some of the damage from high fat diets (Trasino)
- Reducing progression of necrotizing enterocolitis (Zampieri)

**Lactobacillus Plantarum**
- Activation of immune system T-regulatory cells, which limit anaphylactic IgE allergic reaction (Yoshida)
- Modulation of immunity, providing protection against Influenza flu virus (Park)
- Protection of immune system killer cell function from effects of aging or gamma radiation (Lee)

- Protects intestinal epithelial cells from DNA damage that causes cancer (Burns)

**Lactobacillus Rhamnosus**
- Reduces production of inflammatory TNF-a in alcohol-induced liver damage (Wang)
- Helps with asthma (Kim)
- Helps prevent bacterial vaginosis in women with surgically-induced menopause (Parma)
- Reduces IBS (Yoon)
- Reduces fussing and crying in pre-term infants (Partty)
- Administered nasally, prevents respiratory viral infections (Tomosada)
- Helps treat and prevent MSRA infections (Sikorska)
- Protects human colonic muscle from LPS-induced inflammatory damage (Ammoscato)
- Prevents viral respiratory infections in pre-term infants (Luoto)
- Suppresses colon cancer-causing enzymes (Verma)

It is clear, to those studying the microbiome, that no single bacteria has the necessary effect of preserving health in all arenas. In fact, there may not even be a *set* or *grouping* of bacteria that can do this but, rather, a much more complex *interplay between different types of bacteria* that provides benefits, and the exact nature of each bacteria may be less important than the relationship *between* them, their synergistic interactions. What we *do* know is that we have no idea.

# What about Parasitic Worms?

*Parasite Immunology* says:
> "The human immune system has been shaped by its relationship with parasitic worms and this may be a necessary requirement for maintaining our immunological health."[71]

Many types of parasitic worms actually seem to have a beneficial effect on the microbiome, contrary to years of scientific thought. Some worms actually decrease inflammatory processes in the body. According to GAPS Protocol,

> When the microbiome is damaged, the parasites are part of the balance. If they are removed, they will grow back as they are needed in the ecosystem. This would be equivalent to finding worms in the rotting compost pile. You can spend a whole day picking them out and putting them in a glass jar, but they will only grow back as they are needed in ecosystem. [72]

Hookworms, tapeworms, and whipworms have been found to re-balance the bacterial microbiome and help control over-reaction of the immune system. When the body is ill, a high helminth (worm) load is usually found, but the new question, is it the cause of the ailment, or the attempted cure of it by the body's intestinal flora and fauna? *BMC Immunology* says,

---

[71] https://www.ncbi.nlm.nih.gov/pmc/articles/PMC1618732/
[72] https://www.nourishingplot.com/2017/05/23/beneficial-worms-and-bacteria-for-a-healthy-microbiome/

"Parasitic helminths have evolved together with the mammalian immune system over many millennia and as such they have become remarkably efficient modulators in order to promote their own survival. Their ability to alter and/or suppress immune responses could be beneficial to the host by helping control excessive inflammatory responses and animal models and pre-clinical trials have all suggested a beneficial effect of helminth infections on inflammatory bowel conditions, MS, asthma and atopy. Thus, helminth therapy has been suggested as a possible treatment method for autoimmune and other inflammatory disorders in humans."[63]

Please do not make the mistake of thinking all worms are beneficial. Most are not but even more important is that for any worms to be beneficial they must exist in a beneficial balance within the body and in their proper location. Any overload, unbalance or location problem is bad, even of the most beneficial worms.

The reason for so many quotes in this section is that this is such a new concept in biological thought, that "parasites" could also possibly be necessary for a healthy gut and immune system, that I allowed the experts to speak for themselves!

# V. YOU HAVE THREE BRAINS[73]

We are used to thinking of the gray matter inside of our heads as THE BRAIN. In fact, you actually have *three (or more)* brains, and two of them interact actively to produce our emotions and thoughts. The three brains are the neurological brain, the alimentary canal (stomach and intestines, or gut), and the spinal cord with its associated nerves. The alimentary canal contains the second largest number of nerve cells in the body, right after the brain! The spinal cord is made up entirely of nerve cells and controls many automatic functions of the body, in addition to coordinating communications between the alimentary canal, the brain, and all of the other sensory and control nerve cells in the body.

The gut-brain and the head-brain communicate via electric signals carried by the spinal brain and by chemical signals carried by the blood. Many of these chemicals are either directly or indirectly-generated by bacteria in the gut. There is strong evidence that the bacteria/brain relationship is a close one, <u>where many emotional decisions, and even some risk-based ones, are actually made by the bacteria and communicated to the entire organism via chemical signals.</u>

The very old sayings of "go with your gut," "I have a gut feeling," "my gut is nervous," and many other sayings like these are, in fact, true. Trusting your gut is trusting your secondary brain and the bacteria that play a large role in that brain.[74] Most of these bacteria send life-sustaining signals that allow the person carrying them to avoid

---
[73] Many women claim that men have a forth brain that they use for all of their thinking. While there is strong evidence for this conjuncture, it is only an urban myth.

extreme risk. There is also strong evidence that bacteria-gut-brain/head-brain interactions may play a role in depression, suicide, and high risk-taking. There is strong evidence that head-brain degenerative diseases, such as Alzheimers, may start, or first be seen, in the gut. There is also evidence that some parasites from the past may have been beneficial and provided protection against a large laundry list of degenerative diseases, such as Crohn's disease.

There is even a new field of study to understand the gut-brain. This is called neurogastroenterology. Michael Gershon, chairman of the Department of Anatomy and Cell Biology at New York–Presbyterian Hospital/Columbia University Medical Center, wrote a book on the subject in 1998 called "The Second Brain" (Harper Collins). [75] In it, he states that the adult male human brain, at an average of 1.5 kg, has **86 billion** neurons and **85 billion** non-neuronal cells.[76] By contrast, the enteric nervous system in humans consists of some **500 million** neurons (including the various types of Dogiel cells); one two-hundredth of the number of neurons in the brain, and five times as many as the **100 million** neurons in the human spinal cord.[77]

---

[74] https://www.scientificamerican.com/article/gut-second-brain/
[75] The Second Brain, ISBN-10: 0060930721, ISBN-13: 978-0060930721
[76] https://www.ncbi.nlm.nih.gov/pmc/articles/PMC2776484/
[77] https://en.wikipedia.org/wiki/Enteric_nervous_system

# **Super Brain (3 combined)**

|  |  |  |
|---|---|---|
| Brain | 86,000 million | 99.3% |
| Gut | 500 million | 0.6% |
| Spinal | 100 million | 0.1% |
| Total | 86,600 million | 100% |

As you can see, the gut contains 600% more nerve cells than the spinal cord, yet people never think about the gut as having a brain! The gut contains more bacteria than nerve cells, so is there any way that these bacteria wouldn't have an effect on them? These are not even all of the nerve cells in your body!

Good bacteria will help you thrive. Bad bacteria will help themselves at your expense, even to the point of affecting your thoughts.

# VI. REFINED SUGAR AND HFCS

I don't want this chapter to be true. Please someone prove me wrong! As much as I want to be wrong, the evidence is what it is. On the other hand, there are some saving graces to be explored.

Refined sugar is sweet, sweet poison. Before you ever have your first taste, your body is already pre-programmed to want it. As it exists in nature, there is not much wrong with it. As refined sugar, we out-smarted ourselves and hurt our bodies. In addition to the pre-programming, there are two other mechanisms that act upon us to make sugar addictive.

Lets start with defining Refined Sugar vs. Raw Sugar. Many people buy raw sugar, thinking it is unrefined. After the juice is squeezed from sugar cane, it is clarified, precipitated, concentrated, and crystallized until all undesired materials have been removed. The result of all of these processes is what is called unrefined raw sugar. I guess all of the processes mentioned are not considered refining. The difference between sugar cane and unrefined sugar is 80%[78] of the material of the plant has been removed. Refined sugar removes an additional 5%, resulting in a concentrated chemical that does not exist naturally in nature, where 85% of the plant material has been removed, resulting in a final product in which only 15% of the plant is preserved.[79]

---

[78] Yudkin, John,"Pure, White, and Deadly", ISBN 978-0-14-312518-1, page32
[79] "Pure, White, and Deadly", page 33.

Table sugar (refined sugar) is also called sucrose. Sucrose is actually a 50/50 mix of two sugars, glucose and fructose. Fructose seems to the part of sugar that produces most of the bad effects for humans.[80] High Fructose Corn Syrup (HFCS) and High Fructose Syrup (HFS – chemically manufactured) are fructose, so they are 50% worse for you than table sugar! Both HFCS and HFS are banned in Europe, but not for any health related reasons. Sugar beet farmers convinced the ECU to ban the substances as competitive with their products.[81] An additional point to consider is that most (but not all) high intensity, non-caloric sweeteners (artificial sweeteners, such as Splenda®) are actually not as harmful for you as fructose!

## **Role of Sugar in the Body**

Now, lets talk about how sugar is used in the human body. First of all, there is deliberate confusion in how the word sugar is used. Sugar is a family of chemicals with many sub-families. The sugar your body wants is glucose. Glucose is not even remotely similar in action to table sugar, which, as we have already discussed, is made of both glucose and fructose. There have been many experiments by many different institutions on the effects of table sugar on humans.

The results of these experiments have been consistent, therefore I refer to one experiment conducted by Dr. Yudkin on 19 young men. A sugar-enriched diet produced an increase in blood triglycerides in all subjects after 2 weeks. In six of the subjects, the additional changes of about 5 lbs of weight gain, an increase of blood insulin, and

---
[80] "Pure, White, and Deadly", page 36
[81] "Pure, White, and Deadly", page 36

an increase in the stickiness of the platelets were observed.[82] The good news is that all of the changes disappeared after 2 weeks of returning to the subject's normal diet. These are frightful results, but the worst is yet to come.

## **Effects of Sugar on the Liver and Gut**

The liver is the chemical factory of the body. It takes in chemicals and makes what is needed. It is also the toxic waste processing center of the body. It takes in, breaks down, and excretes many toxic substances. If something goes wrong with the liver, the results are body-wide!

When fructose enters the liver, the liver doesn't know what to do with it, so it generates fat, which is stored in both the blood stream and the tissues of the liver. This fat raises the blood triglicerides, but it also causes *Alanine Aminotransferase (ALT) enzymes* to increase in the blood. They are used to measure liver function and damage by increasing in quantity when tissue damage occurs for *any* reason. When the liver is damaged, it releases ALT into the bloodstream as a sort of red flag.[83] In addition, the increase of fat cells tells the body's cells to not burn any sugar, either turning it into more fat or excreting it through the bowels, because the body is in storage mode! This causes a loss of energy/stamina and can cause mood changes, along with 45 minute sugar highs followed by energy crashes and sugar cravings.[84]

---

[82] "Pure, White, and Deadly", Pages 111, 112
[83] www.webmd.com/digestive-disorders/alanine-aminotransferase-alt#1
[84] "That Sugar Film", staring Damon Gameau (2015)

You may *think* that you are not eating sugar but, in fact, sugar has been hidden in almost all processed foods, with the exception of no-sugar-added foods. It is also prevalent in low-fat, processed foods. To get a good idea of how to avoid sugar in your diet, watch the movie "That Sugar Film," by Damon Gameau (2015).

Another dynamic effect of sugar is on the lining of the stomach. I quote from "Pure, White and Deadly";

> "Large amounts of sugar, however, especially if taken in concentrated form on an otherwise empty stomach, will be an irritant. You can actually see the irritation happening if you put a gastroscope into somebody's stomach, which allows you to see the stomach lining. If you now get the subject to swallow a moderately strong sugar solution – the equivalent, say, of four or five lumps in a cup of coffee – you can watch the mucous membrane turn red and angry as the irritant sugar reaches it."[85]

## Biome Changes Due to Sugar

According to the Genetics Department at the University of Utah, "several studies have turned up evidence linking obesity to the microbiome:

- A diet high in fat, sugar, and simple carbs is bad for the "healthy" gut microbes that keep us thin while it encourages the growth of "unhealthy" microbes that make us obese.
- Obese individuals harbor microbes that are better at extracting energy from food, as well as microbes that signal the body to store energy as fat.

---
[85] "Pure, White, and Deadly", page 170

- Bacteria transplanted from overweight mice to thin mice make the thin mice gain weight. "[86]

## **How Hormones Change Due to Sugar**

Sugar can have a profound effect on certain chemicals in the body, one of which is the hormone called insulin. Insulin is secreted by the pancreas in order to turn dietary substances into glucose for the brain and heart to use. Too much sugar, however, can wreak havoc on the carefully-balanced systems of the body. Here is one way in which it can affect us on a molecular level:

> "When insulin spikes, typically after a meal high in sugar, this can lead to lower levels of an important protein known as sex hormone binding globulin (SHBG). SHBG binds excess estrogen and testosterone in the blood, but when it's low, these hormone levels increase. Insulin also increases the production of testosterone, which is then converted into even more estrogen by fat tissue in the belly. [87]

This unbalancing of the ratio of hormones in the body that affect our moods can cause us to become irritable, insomniac, and contribute to anxiety. The best thing we can do is to avoid simple sugars, like sucrose and fructose, and concentrate on eating more complex carbohydrates, fiber, protein, and good fats, which actually cause us to *spend*

---

[86] Genetic Science Learning Center, "The Microbiome And Disease", http://learn.genetics.utah.edu/content/ microbiome/ disease/

[87] https://www.womenshealthnetwork.com/ hormonalimbalance/ hormonal-imbalance-caused-by-sugar.aspx

some energy in order to digest them in a way that simple sugars don't.

> "Also, be sure to include lots of cruciferous vegetables in your diet, like Brussels sprouts, broccoli, cabbage and kale for added hormone balancing."[76]

This provides lots of fiber for your body to work on and keeps the simple sugars to a minimum.

## **Identification of Sugars Hidden in Foods**

The Health Science Academy[88] has identified 65 alternative names used for sugar in the processed food industry. They are presented in the chart on the next page. If any of these appear in the first *four* ingredients on a package, you know you're getting a gutload of sugar!

The exception to that rule is "starch", which may or may not be sugar but, in all cases, *is* a carbohydrate that easily converts into sugar within the body. Therefore, if you see "rich starch", "corn starch", or "potato starch", these are all simple starches that convert readily into sugars.

---

[88] https://thehealthsciencesacademy.org/

| | | |
|---|---|---|
| *Agave nectar | *Dextrose | *Maltodextrin |
| *Agave syrup | *Diastase | *Maltotroise |
| *Barbados sugar | *Diastatic malt | *Maltose |
| *Barley malt | *Ethyl maltol | *Mannitol |
| *Beet sugar | *Evap. cane juice | *Maple syrup |
| *Brown Sugar | *Free-flowing brown sugars | *Molasses |
| *Buttered syrup | *Fructose | *Muscovado |
| *Cane crystals | *Fruit juice | *Panocha |
| *Cane juice | *Fruit juice conc.. | *Powdered sugar |
| *Cane sugar | *Galactose | *Raw sugar |
| *Caramel | *Glucose | *Refiner's syrup |
| *Carob syrup | *Glucose solids | *Rice syrup |
| *Castor sugar | *Golden syrup | *Sorbitol |
| *Corn syrup | *Granulated sugar | *Sorghum syrup |
| *Corn sweetener | *Grape sugar | *Starch |
| *Confectioner's sugar | *High fructose corn syrup | *Sucrose |
| *Corn syrup solids | *Honey | *Syrup |
| *Cryst. fructose | *Icing sugar | *Table sugar |
| *Date sugar | *Invert sugar | *Treacle |
| *Dehydrated cane juice | *Lactose | *Tubinado sugar |
| *Demerara sugar | *Malt | *Yellow sugar |
| *Dextran | *Malt syrup | |

# VII. HUMAN MICROBIOME VS. FERTILIZERS AND POISONS

To a great extent, we treat our body as a garden. There are many historical references as such, and they are true. We constantly add fertilizers and poisons to our body that affect the microorganisms that create our health. Some of these poisons are strange, in that they are beneficial and harmful at the same time. One example is sugar. Sugar is a preservative which kills certain bacteria; however, is it also a fertilizer that enhances some bacteria. The problem is not sugar, but how we consume it and the quantities in which we consume it. In general, white sugar and high fructose corn syrup enhance microorganisms that are not beneficial. Fructose is especially damaging, as we have touched upon before.

When everything is in balance, we can ingest a great deal of poison without harm, but when things are *not* in balance, and the balance is toward loss of health, then even minor poisons, such as nightshades, can have an ill effect.

How does this work and what can we do about it? To a certain extent, we can not avoid many of the poisons without a great deal of work and expense. *Manufactured foods* contain preservatives, which are poison to bacteria. Industrial farming uses *glyphosate (Roundup®)*, which is a strong poison to beneficial bacteria. Many of our foods, such as *Nightshade*-family tomatoes, potatoes, peppers, and eggplants, contain minor poisons as well.

All of this together would not cause us harm usually, except that our food has been industrialized and regulated in ways that cause harm to the human organism. For example, most dietary fiber has been removed from modern, first-world diets. When you combine poisons with the starvation of the beneficial bacterial in the gut by eliminating fiber, the effect is easy to understand. The strange thing is that, even with a heavy poison load, it may still be possible to bring back the beneficial bacteria in as little as 24 hours! The way to do that is by fertilization, using the preferred food of dietary fiber, while removing the most egregious poisons.

## **Chemical Poisons in the Diet**

The modern food industry has "fiddled" with our food until some of it is barely worthy of the name. Food should be nourishing and healthy, but it has been filled with so much poison and had so much of its nutritive value stripped away that we humans end up eating worse food than our own pets! This has resulted in a culture of obesity, with overall health declining at a rapid pace, not only due to sugar, but to other substances that affect one or more of the "brains" of the body.

It would be best for all involved if everyone knew which additives are the worst for the body, and why. To that purpose, here is a list of chemicals our food has been modified with:

- Monosodium Glutamate (MSG)--classified as an excitotoxin, causing brain lesions, obesity, and damage to the hypothalamus[78]

- Artificial sweeteners (aspartame, sucralose)—excitotoxins, affect the nervous system, alters gut flora[89],worsens IBS[90]
- BHA & BHT—potential endocrine disruptor. Has lung, liver, kidney, thyroid affects.[91]
- Sodium Nitrate or Nitrite—unites with amines in meat to cause cancer[92]
- Recombinant Bovine Growth Hormone (rBGT)--links to cancer, early onset puberty, contains insulin-like growth factor, possible diabetogenic.[93]
- Synthetic trans-fat—carcinogen, decreased immune function, diabetagenic, worsens heart disease[94]
- Artificial flavors and colors—grab-bag of chemicals that can cause brain damage, cancer, or affect the microbiome.[84]
- Round-up (glyphosate)--causes imbalance of good/bad bacteria in gut, leading to leaky bowel syndrome and autoimmune disorders.[95]

As you can see, additives can cause the body to swing out of balance as the microbiome is challenged and the brains

---

[89] https://www.globalhealingcenter.com/natural-health/6-dangerous-excito-toxins/

[90] https://articles.mercola.com/sites/articles/archive/2013/12/30/ worst-food-ingredients.aspx

[91] https://www.scientificamerican.com/article/bha-and-bht-a-case-for-fresh/

[92] http://healthyeating.sfgate.com/sodium-nitrate-vs-sodium-nitrite-9064.html

[93] https://www.globalhealingcenter.com/natural-health/8-shocking-facts-bovine-growth-hormone/

[94] https://articles.mercola.com/sites/articles/archive/2013/12/30/ worst-food-ingredients.aspx

[95] https://www.drperlmutter.com/pesticides-damage-microbiome/

of the body are compromised. New legislation may be required to bring our food industries back to a place of nutritional value and balance.

# Gut Bacteria: Friend Or Foe?

One of the things that I fear is that people will read this book and go away with the misconception that all bacteria is good for you! That would be a fatal mistake. There is a reason that antibiotics has brought a big improvement to human and animal health and that reason is that there is more stuff out there that will kill you than there is stuff that will enhance your life.

Knowing the difference between the good stuff and the bad stuff is what all the research is about. The truth is that microbiome treatments go back thousands of years with ancient Chinese Traditional Medicine, but we *still* really have no idea what we are doing.

Human modification of the biome, using scientific methods and an actual understanding of what we are doing, is incomplete. This field of study will be one of the most important, fruitful, and life enhancing of the next 100 years, but we are only at the beginning.

Having said that, there are safe ways to modify the biome. Dietary fiber, along with the general plan presented in this book, will give the body the needed input to modify the biome on its own.

## VIII. SPECIAL FOODS BEYOND FIBER

What would your opinion be if I told you there are special foods that can help your gut and your overall health? I don't think you would be surprised. Of course, the general opinion is that anything strong enough to enhance health could also damage health through side effects. If I *then* told you that this food was as nutritious as oatmeal and so safe that, at one time, it was a traditional food fed to infants to help them wean off of mother's milk? Would you believe me? No? You should. Our modern diets are so processed that we have forgotten many of our traditional foods. Just like dietary fiber.

# Slippery Elm

The food that I am talking about is Slippery Elm. You may know it as something you take when you have a cold. It is a powerful herbal ingredient, but it is also a nutritious food. The specific form of Slippery Elm I am writing about is Ulmus rubra; U. fulva of the family *Ulmaceae*.

Here is an extract from the book, "School of Natural Healing, 25th Anniversary Edition" by Dr. John R. Christopher:

> "It is also wonderful for the elderly or convalescents; it possesses as much nutrition as oatmeal, though it is much easier on the system, and is an excellent sustaining food." The book goes on to describe it as a "remedy in all cases of weakness, pulmonary complaints, stomach inflammation, lung

hemorrhage, absorbing noxious gases and neutralizing acidity in the stomach."[96]

You can make this marvelous food for yourself. It's easy.

# **Honey**

There is one other ingredient that is used to make what we call "Slippery Elm Balls", and that is honey. Honey has a good side and a bad side. In this case, the good side outweighs the bad side, since it is being used for a specific purpose, not in excess, or just as a sweetener. Honey is made up monosaccharides; specifically, the same sugars found in table sugar, fructose and glucose. Honey may or may not contain a few other sugars. While the glucose adds calories, it is easily assimilated and burned by the body. Fructose is the evil sibling. In this case, we will ignore it because honey has other properties that we want and *that* makes up for the fructose!

**Warning: Infants should *never* eat honey.** It can kill them.[97] Never collect honey yourself because, depending upon the plants used by the bees, the honey could cause something called Mad Honey Intoxication, which can kill you.[98] Excess honey consumption can cause serious medical problems and can *also* kill you. In this recipe, we will *not* be using enough to cause problems.

The benefits of honey are harder to understand. It has been used for medical purposes for thousands of years (mentioned as medicine in Ancient Egypt) and anything

---
[96] School of Natural Healing, ISBN 1-879436-01-9, Page 366
[97] https://en.wikipedia.org/wiki/Honey
[98] https://en.wikipedia.org/wiki/Honey

that has proven itself by the test of time must have benefits or people would not do it. This is, of course, not scientific. From a scientific view point, honey has been proven to kill food-borne pathogens, such as E. coli, Salmonella, Staphylococcus aureus, and Pseudomonas aeruginosa.[99] Honey has not been *scientifically proven* to have the same effect after eating, but I believe the main reason is that no one has looked.

You should also understand that there is *medical* honey, which is used for wound care, and there are other honeys that are used by herbalists for various ailments. In this case, they use specific honeys gathered from specific plants and not generic or blended honey. We will be using generic honey, since it contains all of the preservation, viscosity, tactical, sweetness, and flavor properties we want for this project. Personally, my opinion is that, when used correctly and in moderation, honey is beneficial.

**Warning**: A great deal of the honey sold in the United States and elsewhere is fake. It is *not* honey at all but honey flavored syrup. This syrup is not only fake but *harmful*. Be aware that very inexpensive honey and, unfortunately, some *expensive* honey, may not be real or a blend of fake and real. Be careful.

There is a great deal more to know about the benefits and drawbacks of honey. This book only deals with what is needed for the specific subject under discussion. I refer you to the Internet and high quality books on the subject for additional information.

---

[99] http://www.webmd.com/diet/features/medicinal-uses-of-honey

# Slippery Elm Honey Balls

I was reminded of Slippery Elm by my friend Eileen Mcaliney, who gave me a gift of home-made Slippery Elm Honey Balls. Not only do they work, but they taste *good*. I had no problem getting an elderly relative to eat one every day. He would never have eaten it otherwise, and he would *never* have taken the capsules. Eileen credits Susan Weed (www.susanweed.com & www.wisewomanuniversity.com) for information on this herbal preparation. See https://m.youtube.com/watch?v=51Bi_6lfla8 for a video on Slippery Elm.

Here is the recipe that Eileen used to make the balls she gave me:

1) Put 1 pound slippery elm bark powder in a bowl.

2) Add an equal amount by weight of honey and knead until you have a thick paste similar to pie dough. If you want to make a small amount, use equal parts of slippery elm and honey by weight.

3) Roll the paste into small balls of around 1-inch in diameter.

4) Roll the balls in dry, slippery elm powder, so they don't stick together, and box.

Eileen credits Monica Jean for the recipe. Video at https://www.youtube.com/watch?v=3XDuFprnEVc&t=7s

# IX. SUMMATION ON FIBER

1. Dietary fiber is critical to the support of the gut's healthy microbiome.
2. The gut's microbiome creates many valuable hormones, can affect thoughts and food cravings, and is an important part of the immune system. The gut actually contains one of a human's three brains, all of which communicate with each other!
3. Common chemicals, such as glyphosate (RoundUp®[100]), can harm your gut's good microbiome. These chemicals are on almost all not-organic foods.
4. Nitrates/Nitrites are common food preservatives used in processed meats that also can harm a good microbiome.
5. Some common foods, such as table sugar, fruit juices, and high fructose corn syrup, support the growth of bad bacteria in the gut, which unbalances the healthy microbiome.
6. In general, foods and chemicals assist either the good or the bad bacteria, but usually do not assist both. The same is true of foods and chemicals which harm the good or bad bacteria, but do not harm both.
7. The safest way to rebuild a damaged microbiome is to eat at least 35 grams of mixed dietary fiber per day, for an adult. This fiber enhances the good bacteria, which can then crowd out the bad bacteria. You can also take high quality probiotics or visit an appropriate doctor, who can apply the gut bacteria more directly.
8. There are good and bad bacteria. The more common problem is one of imbalance. Imbalance can cause bacteria that would normally not be harmful to act in harmful ways. Generally, imbalance and lack of biodiversity is the real problem with the gut's microbiome.

[100] ROUNDUP® is a trademark by Monsanto Company, Saint Louis, MO, 63167.

9. The most important thing to know is that an imbalance of the gut's microbiome can be corrected by you. You do this by avoiding certain chemicals, such as glyphosate, preservatives, and sugar, while eating probiotics, live fermented foods, and enough mixed dietary fiber to feed the good bacteria.

10. Even if you can not eat "clean" foods, you can eat dietary fiber, and encourage the "good" bacteria to multiply and crowd out the "bad" bacteria.

Many of these problems came into existence because modern developed countries removed dietary fiber from processed foods, then removed good fats and replaced them with bad sugars. They also replaced good, balanced fats with low quality, bad fats that are unbalanced.

How could we be healthy when we removed the fiber that was keeping us healthy, and then added poisons? Make no mistake; anything that is a poison to our microbiome is a poison to us.

# X. BONUS MATERIAL

# Mother Dirt

I learned about the microbiome of the skin from a book which discussed a product from a company called Mother Dirt[101]. This fit right in with my thirst for knowledge about the microbiome of the entire body. It also fit with some of my past experiences. I once met a doctor from Bulgaria. She was a Doctor of Cosmetology. I told her that I didn't understand her title because a Cosmetologist was a title in the United States, but it was someone who sold cosmetics. She was shocked and went on to explain what she did. Her profession is a medical doctor who diagnoses a patient by looking at them. She is especially careful to examine the skin because "all the problems of the body are exhibited on the skin". What she does is similar to what a family doctor does in the United States but, because they don't have all the fancy diagnostic equipment, they use a different paradigm.

This made me think, if the outside reflects the inside, then does the outside *affect* the inside? Is it a two-way street? Can improvement of our skin's health affect our internal health? This is yet to be proven, but I would be surprised if it is not true.

This experience made me instantly understand the importance of the microbiome of the skin and what the Mother Dirt company is attempting to do, which is nothing short of correcting the skin microbiome with direct application of one specific bacteria that makes the skin a

---

[101] MOTHERDIRT is a trademark of AOBIOME.

much healthier (and beautiful) place for beneficial bacteria to grow, while suppressing bad or imbalanced bacteria.

I purchase a single bottle of the Mother Dirt product "AO+MIST" and was so impressed that I purchased a subscription for 1 bottle every 3 months. As I continued to use the product and saw the benefits for myself, I expanded the use of the product and changed my subscription from 1 bottle every 3 months to 1 bottle every 2 months. I can see even that changing in the future.

Here is information from the label of the bottle:

> INGREDIENTS: Water, Nitrosomonas Eutropha (live, cultured, Ammonia-Oxidizing Bacteria), disodium phosphate, magnesium chloride (natural salts). FOR TOPICAL USE ONLY.

They continue with an explanation of the product:

> Formulated for compatibility with the skin's natural microbiome. Learn more at biomefriendly.com. Questions: hello@motherdirt.com

**Their website is www.motherdirt.com**

# GrainFields

There are a lot of brands of probiotics on the market. I feel that, at one time or another, I have purchased all of them. Very few seem to have any detectable effect on me. The expensive ones had the same effect as the inexpensive ones; nothing.

While visiting my distributor in Brooklyn, they handed me a bottle of Grainfields probiotic liquid. They import it from Australia. I did not expect much, but it actually had a noticeable benefit. When I gave it to elderly relatives, it had a pronounced beneficial effect. While I have not used probiotics on a daily basis, I now have a favorite and it is Grainfields.

Grainfields is made from a blend of malt, oats, maize, rice, wheat, millet and buckwheat. I don't like using grains that contain gluten, but I was unofficially told that the gluten is digested by the bacteria and would qualify as gluten-free, if they could afford the costs of making that legal claim. I am gluten-intolerant and have not experienced any problems using the product. However, buyer beware. Decide for yourself or ask your medical doctor.

The bacteria Grainfields uses to make their product are certified organic, non-GMO, and non-GE. They claim that the strains used are all present in a healthy, human digestive system and are, therefore, good for anyone who is missing these strains. The strains used are:

- Lactobacillus Acidophilus
- Bifidus (Bifidobacterium)
- Lactobacillus casi

- Lactobacillus helveticus
- Lactobacillus bulgaricus
- Lactobacillus leichmannii
- Lactobacillus caucasicus
- Lactobacillus lactis
- Lactobacillus fermenti
- Lactobacillus brevis
- Lactobacillus plantarum
- Lactobacillus delbreukii

with healthy yeast strains:
- Saccharomyces boulardi
- Saccharomyces cerevisiae.

One of the reasons why I believe that some of the probiotics I've used in the past had no effect is because the stomach acid probably killed the bacteria before they could work. The yeasts used in this product are proven to be acid-resistant and are known to provide beneficial enzymes and B vitamins as a by-product, in addition to their ability to kill Candida. Candida infections can be common.

**www.grainfieldsusa.com**
Grainfields USA LLC /The Essence of Life®
451 6th Ave. Brooklyn, NY. 11215

Grainfields@icloud.com OR r.grainfieldsusa@gmail.com
Phone:1-718-788-8783    Cell 347-236-6334

Wholesale inquiries welcome ~ Rebecca Grainfields

# DIETARY FIBER BOOKS IN MY LIBRARY

The following books on dietary fiber are in my personal library and have strongly influenced the writing of this book. Some of these books may be out of print and only available from libraries.

This is not all of the books in my library on the subject matter of dietary fiber. Some of the books may not appear to be on fiber at all but neither the less are related to the subject matter. The books are not listed in any order. I found them all worth while and recommend reading them.

Atkins, Michael," Good Gut", 2015. ISBN 9781522942368

Axe, Dr. Josh, 'Eat Dirt', 2016. ISBN: 978-0-06-243364-0

Brumback, Roger A., MD; Brumback, Mary H.. BS, Rph, "The Dietary Fiber Weight Control Handbook" 1989. ISBN: 1-4196-3594-8

Campbell, Kristina, "The Well-Fed Microbiome Cookbook", 2016. ISBN: 978-1-62315-736-4

Chutkan, Robynne, "The Microbiome Solution", 2015. ISBN: 978-0-399-57350-7

Collen, Alanna, "10% Human," 2015. ISBN: 978-0-06-134598-1

Curtis, Sky, "The Fecal Transplant Guidebook", 2013. ISBN-13: 9780991952021

Elkins, Rita, M.H., "Fiber Facts", 1999. ISBN: 1-58054-068-6

Farris, Russel; Marin, Per, M.D., PhD., "The Potbelly Syndrome", 2006. ISBN-13: 978-1-59120-058-1

Kellman, Raphael, MD, "The Microbiome Diet", 2014. ISBN: 978-0-7382-1820-5

Kritchevsky, David & Bonfield, Charles, Editors, "Dietary Fiber in Health and Disease",1995. ISBN: 0-9624407-6-0

Kritchevsky, David; Bonfield, Charles; and Anderson, James W., Editors, "Dietary Fiber Chemistry, Physiology and Health Effects," 1990. ISBN: 0-306-43310-9

Lorenzani, Shirley S., Ph.D., "Dietary Fiber," 1988. ISBN: 0-87983-479-X

Madar, Zecharia, and Odes, H. Selwyn, "Progress in Biochemical Pharmacology Volume 24 – Dietary Fiber Research", 1990. ISBN: 3-8055-5043-X

Matthews, Richard, DC, DACNB, FACFN, "The Symbiont Factor," 2014. ISBN: 9781500553944

Nozawa, Yashi, "Fecal Transplant Early History of FMT," 2015. ISBN-13: 978-1507834633

Prosky, Leon, and Devries, Jonathan, "Controlling Dietary Fiber In Food Products", 1992. ISBN: 0-442-00239-4

Spiller, Gene A., Ed., "CRC Handbook Of Dietary Fiber in Human Nutrition 3rd Edition", 2001. ISBN: 0-8493-2387-8

Vaccariello, Liz / Rodale Press, "Prevention Fiber Up Slim Down Cookbook", 2008. ISBN-13: 978-1594868016

Velasquez-Manoff, Moises, "An Epidemic of Absence," 2012. ISBN: 978-1-4391-9938-1

Vahouny, George V., and Kritchevsky, David, "Dietary Fiber in Health and Disease,"1982. ISBN: 0-306-40926-7

Walker, Norman W., D.Sc., Ph.D., "Colon Health", 1995 ISBN: 0-89019-069-0

Yudkin, John, "Pure, White and Deadly," 1986. ISBN: 978-0-14-312518-1

# Other Books That I Am Reading

This is a list of a few of the books that I am reading at the moment. I enjoy reading and decided to share a few of the titles that I thought you might find interesting. This is not an endorsement of the books, their contents or authors. It is only a list of what I am actually reading. All of these books are available on amazon.com and other booksellers.

### "Vitamin K2 and the Calcium Paradox"
Kate Rheaume-Bleue, B.Sc., N.D.
Extract from the back cover:
*Are you taking calcium or vitamin D? This book could save your life!*
*Learn the secret to avoiding osteoporosis and heart disease. Millions of people take vitamin D and calcium supplements for bone health. But new research shows that this actually increases the risk of heart attack and stroke because extra calcium builds up in the arteries – the Calcium Paradox. The secret to keeping bones strong and*

*arteries clear is vitamin K2, a little-known super-nutrient that humans once consumed in abundance and that has been ignored by scientists for almost 70 years.*

### "The Magnesium Miracle"
Carolyn Dean, M.D., N.D.
Extract from the back cover:
*Magnesium is an essential nutrient, indispensable to your health and well-being. By adding this mineral to your diet, you are guarding against – and helping to alleviate – such threats as heart disease, stroke, osteoporosis, diabetes, depression, arthritis, and asthma. But despite magnesium's numerous benefits, many Americans remain dangerously deficient.*

### "The Big Fat Surprise"
Nina Teicholz
Extract from the fly-cover
*In this captivating, vibrant, and convincing narrative, based on a nine year long investigation, Teicholz shows how the misinformation about saturated fats took hold in the scientific community and the public imagination, and how recent findings have overturned these beliefs.*

# GLOSSARY [102] [103] [104]

**A**

**Acetate**—derivative of acetic acid. Used as a counter-irritant and a reagent in chemical reactions.

**ADA**—Americans with Disabilities Act regulates compliance with regulations protecting the disabled.

**Alanine Aminotransferase (ALT) enzymes**—an enzyme that converts amino acid L-Alanine to L-glutamate

**Alimentary**—organ system that includes the mouth, esophagus, stomach, intestines, and anus, used to digest food and eliminate wastes from the body.

**Amylose**—a polysaccharide chain that is found in some starches

**Anaphylactic**—acute, unhealthy reaction to a substance that was previously encountered. Reactions can range from mere itching to shock and death.

**Antimicrobial agents**—any substance that can destroy or prevent spread of microbes

**Apnea**—absence of breathing, especially during sleep.

**Aspartame**—artificial sweetener, irritates nervous system and stomach lining, alters gut flora

**ATP**—a neurotransmitter, also an energy-transfer molecule in the cell

**Atherosclerosis**—so-called "hardening of the arteries" by fat deposits on blood vessel walls

**Autoimmune**—body's immune system begins to attack the tissues of the body for no discernible reason.

---

[102] Courtesy of http://www.online-medical-dictionary.org/
[103] Courtesy of medical-dictionary.thefreedictionary.com/
[104] Courtesy of en.wikipedia.org/wiki/

## B

**Bacteria**—one-celled organisms, can be either beneficial or malignant to the human body

**Bacillus coagulans**—a beneficial bacteria found in the gut, rarely pathogenic, aids with food digestion.

**BHA/BHT**—food additive that is an endocrine disruptor

**Bifidobacterium**-- infantis, animalis, breve, bifidum—beneficial bacteria found in the gut, aids with food digestion.

**Bile**—created by the liver, it assists in digestion of fats in the duodenum.

**Biomarker**—something biological used to identify or measure its presence in another substance

**BMI**—Basal Metabolic Index—a measure of body fat based on height/weight.

**Butyrate**—a short-chain fatty acid used in flavoring extracts and perfumes

## C

**Candida**—yeast-like fungus normally found in alimentary canal, but can overgrow and cause problems

**Carbohydrate**—a combination of carbon, hydrogen, and oxygen; a food source of energy for the body, such as sugars and starches. Can be changed into fats in large quantities. Polysaccharides are also carbs.

**Cardiovascular**—pertaining to the heart and its blood vessels.

**Cellulose**—carbohydrates that form the structures of plants. Polysaccharide. Dietary fiber.

**Chitin**—a polysaccharide that makes up insect shells and certain fungi. Similar to cellulose.

**Cholesterol**—found in animal fats and oils, that makes up most of the body cell walls, can create stones. Usually created by the body's liver.

**Circadian rhythm**—cycle between day and night. A 24-hour cycle

**Colonocytes**—the inside-most cell of the lining of the large intestine.

**Clostridium difficile**—bacteria found in human feces. Can cause illness if it infects other organs or in case of overgrowth.

**Colon**—the large intestine of the human alimentary canal. Aids in digestion and re-absorption of water from stool.

**Colitis**—inflammation of the large intestine due to infection or overgrowth of bacteria. May cause diarrhea, cramping, and pain.

**Constipation**—an inability to pass stool due to low motility, or blockage, of the large intestine/sigmoid colon/rectum.

**Contrabiotic**--blocks mucosal adherence and relocation of bad bacteria in the colon and may diminish intestinal inflammation,

**Cristae**-- folds on the inside wall of the mitochondria

**Crohn's Diseases**—form of chronic inflammation involving the distal small and complete large intestine, with ulcers, narrowing of the passage, and flu-like symptoms.

**Cruciferous vegetables**—broccoli, cabbage, and other green, leafy vegetables, part of the mustard family

**Cytoplasm**—gel-like substance inside cell walls, also called protoplasm. Contains organelles like mitochondria.

# **D**

**Dendritic cell**—a branch of a nerve cell that carries impulses to another place.

**Diverticulitis**—inflammation of a pocket in the intestine (diverticulum) that may cause pain and rupture if filled with feces.

**Disaccharides**—sugar created by two monosaccharides, such as lactose or sucrose.

**DNA**—genetic material that acts as the blueprint for reproduction of a cell.

**Duodenal Ulcer**—an inflammatory ulcer of the mucous membrane in the high small intestine.

**Dysbiosis**—unhealthy, unbalanced biome, such as when antibiotics are used.

## E

**Endogenous**—internally produced by an organism, tissue, or cell

**Enzyme**—a compound that serve to initiate a biochemical reaction.

## F

**Fauna**—animal life, includes microbes.

**Fiber, water-insoluble**—fiber that doesn't dissolve in water and maintains its original properties.

**Fiber, water-soluble**—fiber that dissolves in water and becomes gel-like

**Fecal transplant**—transplant of healthy fecal matter from one human gut biome to another

**Feces**—waste matter of the body, made up of dead microbes, fiber, undigested food, dead cells

**Fibromyalgia**—inflammatory disorder of the nervous and muscle tissues, causing pain, stiffness.

**Flatulence**—gaseous by-products of digestion, emitted by the anus.

**Flora**—vegetable life, including fungi and yeast

**Fructans**—polymer of fructose molecules

**Fructo-oligosaccharide**—fructan with a short chain length

**Fungicide**—a substance that kills fungi or fungal spores

## G

**Gastroesophageal reflux**—the weakening of the cardiac sphincter of the stomach, allowing gastric contents to move up the esophagus under pressure

**Gastrointestinal**—pertaining to the stomach and intestinal tract

**Gelatin**—a solution of soluble fiber and water

**Gestational Diabetes**—type II diabetes that occurs because of pregnancy; may be temporary.

**Glucose**—single sugar, used as fuel for all tissues of the body.

**Glycoside**—plant-derived component of a drug or poison

**Glyphosate**—RoundUp, a pesticide that can alter the gut microbiome, found on plants

**GMO**—Genetically Modified Organism.

**Goodbelly**—a probiotic drink containing lactobacillus plantarum

**Grainfields**—probiotic supplement, provides yeast for microbiome growth

**Gut**—collective of stomach, intestines, sigmoid colon, & rectum.

## **H**

**Helminths**—worms. Some, such as hookworms, tapeworms, and whipworms, can be beneficial to the gut biome. Others are parasitic.

**Hemicellulose**—polysacchaarides which make up the cell walls of plants.

**Herbicides**—chemical substances that kill plants.

**Herbivores**—plant-eating animals.

**Hexose**—simple sugars containing six carbon atoms, such as glucose and fructose.

**HFCS**—High Fructose Corn Syrup. Contains glucose and fructose polymers. A high-caloric sweetener

**HFS**—A high-caloric sweeter like HFCS.

**Hyperglycemia**—elevated level of sugar in the blood, usually found in diabetes mellitus

**Hypertension**—persistently elevated blood pressure, usually above 140/100.

# I

**Immune-modulating**—natural, non-allergic substances that support the immune system.

**Immunoglogulin E**—Antibody found in mammals, fights parasites.

**Inositol**—multiple-alcohol sugar

**Inflammation**----immune response of the body to attacking organisms. Redness, heat, pain, itching may be part of the response.

**TNF-a**—tumor necrosis factor alpha, a protein involved in acute inflammation reaction

**Insulin resistance**—condition in which pancreatic cells don't respond to the hormone insulin, resulting in hyperglycemia.

**Inulin**—a natural carbohydrate that stores sugar in the body.

**Irritable Bowel Syndrome**—a group of symptoms indicating irritation in bowel, including pain, change in bowel habits, cramping. There is no apparent disease process.

**Isoflavones**—also called phytoestrogens. Estragenic-like substance found in plants.

## K

**Kombucha**—fermented, slightly carbonated black or green tea drink. Produced by fermenting tea using beneficial bacteria and yeast

## L

**Lactobacillus**-- plantarum, acidophilus, rhamnosus, paracasei, casei, fermentum—a form of bacteria that converts sugar to lactic acid in the gut.

**Lactulose**—non-absorbable sugar used for constipation and to treat liver toxicity

**Laparoscopic**—examination of the inside of the abdomen using a thin viewing device called a laparoscope.

**Leaky gut**—a condition of increased permeabulity (leaking) of the intestinal wall, causing inflammation throughout the body.

**Leukocytes**—cells of the immune system that protect against disease and parasites.

**Lignan**—one of the phytoestrogens that also acts as an antioxidant.. usually found in nut, seeds, grains, some beans and fruits, and cruciferous vegetables.

**LPS-induced inflammation**—lipopolysaccharides found in tobacco and some dusts can cause inflammation and damage in the respiratory system.

## M

**Metabolic syndrome**—a cluster of symptoms that are associated with cardiovascular disease and type II Diabetes. They include obesity, high blood pressure and serum triglycerides and low high-density lipoprotein.

**Microbes**—a microscopic organism, may be single-celled or a colony

**Microbiome**—the flora and fauna of a particular system; in this case, the gut of a human being

**Monoshccharides**—simple sugars, most basic carbohydrate. Used to build more complex sugars. Glucose, fructose, galactose are simple sugars.
**Monomeric**—single-named.
**MRSA**-- methicillin-resistant Staphylococcus aureus—a microbe found mostly in soil and are different from S. Aureus. Resistant to penicillin-related antibiotics. May be fatal.
**MSG**—a flavoring agent, also a neurotoxin
**Mucosa**—mucous membrane, lining the nose, mouth, eyes, and genitals .
**Myocardial infarction**—commonly known as a "heart attack"; damage done to the heart from a blocked vessel

## N

**Necrotizing enterocolitis**—severe inflammation of the small and large intestines, leading to death of tissue.
**Neurogastroenterology**—the study of the interactions of the brain, nervous system, and the gut.
**Neurological**—relating to the nervous system.
**Neurons**—cells in the nervous system that transmit electrical impulses throughout the body

## O

**Obesity**—excess body fat which may have an adverse effect on health as determined by BMI
**Occam's razor**—Theory that "the simplest explanation is usually the best."
**Oligosaccharides**—a sugar polymer containing a small number of simple sugars.

## P

**Pathogenic**—injurious to health

**Pectin**—a structural polysaccharide found in the cell walls of plants. A dietary fiber.

**Pentose**—a sugar containing 5 carbon atoms, such as ribose and xylose.

**Pesticides**—chemical substances that kill "pests", such as weeds, insects, worms, rats, mice, microbes, etc.

**Phytic acid**—the principle storage form of phosphorus in bran, seeds, cereals, and grains.

**Platelets**—a blood cell that stops bleeding by clotting off injured blood vessel walls.

**Polydextrose**—synthetic polymer of glucose; a soluble fiber.

**Polymer**—a large molecule made up of many repeating sub-units bound together to create things like plastics and resins.

**Polysaccharide**—a carbohydrate made up of long chains of simple sugars.

**Polyuronides**—a polysaccharide made up of uronic acid molecules, may have other simple sugars or not.

**Prebiotic**—substances that promote the growth or activity of beneficial microbes

**Probiotic**—microbes that claim to provide health benefits

**Preservatives**—chemical that lengthens the shelf life of products by preventing decomposition of its components.

**Propionate**—common short-chain fatty acid produced by the gut in response to indigestible fiber.

**Pseudomonas aeruginosa**—a multi-drug-resistant pathogen that attacks during other illnesses.

## R

**rBGT**—recombinant Bovine Growth Hormone—a diabetogenic hormone, with links to cancer. It promotes milk production in cows.

**Resistant starch**—R1, R2, R3 are fermented by the gut microbiota, which produce short-chain fatty acids.

**Rheumatological**—pertaining to rheumatic diseases, usually of the joints and bones.

**Rhinovirus**—common cold virus. "rhino" refers to the nose.

**Ribosomes**—organelles in the cell that are responsible for protein synthesis.

**RNA**—a polymer required to code, decode, regulate, and express genes in the cell.

**Roughage**—insoluble fiber.

## S

**Saccharide**—a sugar molecule

**Salmonella**—enterobacterium that causes vomiting and diarrhea when ingested. Found in poorly-stored food. Also known as "food poisoning"

**SCFA**--Short Chain Fatty Acids--fatty acids with 2-6 carbon atoms. Also referred to as "volatile fatty acids"

**SHBG**--Sex Hormone Binding Globulin--a glycoprotein that binds to androgen and estrogen.

**Slippery elm**—the "slippery" inner bark of the tree is used as a fiber to regulate the bowels.

**Sodium nitrate/nitrite**—food preservative that causes cancer

**Streptococcus thermophilus**—a lactic-acid microbe that ferments milk products.

**Sucralose**—artificial sweetener, irritates the nervous system and stomach lining and alters gut flora

**Symbiotes**—symbiotic bacteria that live with other organisms to their mutual advantage.

## T
**T-cell**—a type of white blood cell that assists in cell-mediated immunity.
**Toxins**—a poison or venom of plant or animal origin which causes disease when present in low doses.

## V
**Vaginosis**—inflammation of the vagina due to overgrowth of bacteria, with foul odor, discharge, itching.
**Vitamin D**—fat-soluble vitamin that assist in absorption of calcium and other vital minerals.
**Vitamin K**—fat-soluble vitamin that is responsible for blood clotting and assists with calcium management.

# ADDITIONAL REFERENCE MATERIAL

Aaccnet.org--DietaryFiber--dietfiber.pdf

Abrams S, Griffin I, Hawthorne K, Liang L, Gunn S, Darlington G, Ellis K (2005). "A Combination Of Prebiotic Short- And Long-Chain Inulin-Type Fructans Enhances Calcium Absorption And Bone Mineralization In Young Adolescents". Am J Clin Nutr. 82 (2): 471–6. PMID 16087995.

Alvarado A, Pacheco-Delahaye E, Hevia P (2001). "Value Of A Tomato Byproduct As A Source Of Dietary Fiber In Rats" (PDF). plant Foods Hum Nutr. 56 (4): 335–48. doi:10.1023/A: 1011855316778. PMID 11678439.

American Association of Cereal Chemists. "The Definition Of Dietary Fiber: Report Of The Dietary Fiber Definition Committee To The Board Of Directors Of The American Association Of Cereal Chemists". Cereal Foods World. 2001; 46:112–26.

Anderson JW, Baird P, Davis RH, et al. (2009). "Health Benefits Of Dietary Fiber". Nutr Rev. 67 (4): 188–205. doi:10.1111/ j. 1753-4887. 2009. 00189.x. PMID 1933 5713.

British Nutrition Foundation, Dietary fibre.

Boerjan, Wout; Ralph, John; Baucher, Marie (2003). "Lignin-Biosynthesis". Annual Review of Plant Biology. 54:519–46. doi:10.1146/annurev.Arplant.54. 031902.134938. PMID14503002.

Brown L, Rosner B, Willett WW, Sacks FM (1999). "Cholesterol-lowering Effects Of Dietary Fiber: A Meta-Analysis". Am J Clin Nutr. 69 (1): 30–42. PMID 9925120.

Burton-Freeman, Britt, Amgen, Incorporated, "Symposium: Dietary Composition and Obesity: Do We Need to Look Beyond Dietary Fat?," Thousand Oaks, CA 91320-1799,

Carey MC, Small DM and Bliss CM. "Lipid Digestion And Absorption." Annual Review of Physiology. 1983.45:651-677.

Cavaglieri CR, Nishiyama A, Fernandes LC, Curi R, Miles EA, Calder PC (August 2003). "Differential Effects Of Short-Chain Fatty Acids On Proliferation And Production Of Pro- And Anti-Inflammatory Cytokines By Cultured Lymphocytes". Life Sciences. 73 (13): 1683–90. doi:10.1016/S0024-3205(03) 00490-9. PMID 12875900.

Codex Alimentarius Commission; Food and Agriculture Organization; World Health Organization. "Report Of The 30th Session Of The Codex Committee On Nutrition And Foods For Special Dietary Uses." ALINORM 9/32/26. 2009 [cited 2012 Mar 27]. Available from: www.codexalimentarius.net/download/report/710/al32_26e.pdf..

Coudray C, Demigné C, Rayssiguier Y (2003). "Effects Of Dietary Fibers On Magnesium Absorption In Animals And Humans". J Nutr. 133 (1): 1–4. PMID 12514257.

Drozdowski LA, Dixon WT, McBurney MI, Thomson AB (2002). "Short-chain Fatty Acids And Total Parenteral Nutrition Affect Intestinal Gene Expression". J Parenter

Enteral Nutr. 26 (3): 145–50. doi: 10.1177/ 0148607 102026003145. PMID 12005453.

Eastwood MA. "The Physiological Effect Of Dietary Fiber: An Update." Annual Review Nutrition, 1992:12 : 19-35

Eastwood MA, Hamilton D (1968). "Studies On The Adsorption Of Bile Salts To Non-Absorbed Components Of Diet". Biochim. Biophys. Acta. 152: 159–166.

Eastwood M, Kritchevsky D (2005). "Dietary Fiber: How Did We Get Where We Are?". Annu Rev Nutr. 25: 1–8. doi: 10.1146/ annurev.nutr. 25.121304. 131658. PMID 16011456.

Eastwood MA, Morris ER (1992). "Physical Properties Of Dietary Fibre That Influence Physiological Function: A Model For Polymers Along The Gastrointestinal Tract". Am J Clin Nutr. 55: 436–442.

Edwards CA, Johnson IT, Read NW. "Do Viscous Polysaccharides Reduce Absorption By Inhibiting Diffusion Or Convection?" Eur J Clin Nutr 1988;42:307-12.

Ewaschuk JB, Dieleman LA (October 2006). "Probiotics And Prebiotics In Chronic Inflammatory Bowel Diseases". World J Gastroenterol. 12 (37):5941–50. PMID 17009391.Archived from the original on 13 September 2008.

FDA/CFSAN A Food Labeling Guide: Appendix C Health Claims, April 2008

Fischer MH, Yu N, Gray GR, Ralph J, Anderson L, Marlett JA. (2004) "The Gel-Forming Polysaccharide Of Psyllium

Husk (Plantago Ovata Forsk)". Carbohydr Res. 2004 Aug 2;339 (11): 2009-17.

Fotiadis, Constantine Iosif Stoidis, Christos Nikolaou; Spyropoulos, Basileios Georgiou; Zografos, Eleftherios Dimitriou (14 November 2008). "Role Of Probiotics, Prebiotics And Synbiotics In Chemoprevention For Colorectal Cancer". World Journal of Gastroenterology. 14. 14 (42): 6454. doi:10.3748/ wjg.14.6453. ISSN 1007-9327. Archived from the original (PDF) on 28 September 2009. Retrieved 22 April 2009.

Food and Drug Administration, "Advisory Letter Concerning Docket No. FDA-2012-N-1210-0132 (see attached PDF)". Regulations.gov. 30 July 2014. Retrieved 22 August 2014.

Food and Nutrition Board, Institute of Medicine of the National Academies (2005). "Dietary Reference Intakes For Energy, Carbohydrate, Fiber, Fat, Fatty Acids, Cholesterol, Protein, And Amino Acids (Macronutrients)". National Academies Press. pp. 380–382.

Friedman G (September 1989). "Nutritional Therapy Of Irritable Bowel Syndrome". Gastroenterol Clin North Am. 18 (3): 513–24. PMID 2553606.

Fuchs CS, Giovannucci EL, Colditz GA, et al. (January 1999). "Dietary Fiber And The Risk Of Colorectal Cancer And Adenoma In Women". N Engl J Med. 340 (3): 169–76. doi:10. 1056/ NEJM 199901213400301. PMID 9895396.

Gallaher, Daniel D. (2006). "Dietary Fiber". Washington, D.C.: ILSI Press. pp. 102–110. ISBN 978-1-57881-199-1.

Gillissen and Eastwood; Eastwood, Martin A. (1995). "Taurocholic Acid Adsorption During Non-Starch Polysaccharide Fermentation: An In Vitro Study". British Journal of Nutrition. 74 (2): 221–227. doi:10.1079/ BJN19950125.

Grabitske, Hollie A.; Slavin, Joanne L. (2009). "Gastrointestinal Effects of Low-Digestible Carbohydrates". Critical Reviews in Food Science and Nutrition. 49 (4): 327–360. doi:10.1080/10408390802067126 PMID 19234944.

Greger JL (July 1999). "Nondigestible Carbohydrates And Mineral Bio-Availability". J Nutr. 129 (7 Suppl):1434S–5S. PMID 10395614.[permanent dead link]

Gropper, Sareen S.; Jack L. Smith; James L. Groff (2008). "Advanced Nutrition And Human Metabolism (5th Ed.)". cengage Learning. p. 114. ISBN 978-0-495-11657-8. Guarner F (April 2005). "Inulin And Oligofructose: Impact On Intestinal Diseases And Disorders". Br J Nutr. 93 Suppl 1: S61–5. Doi: 10.1079/ BJN20041345. PMID 15877897.

Harvard School of Public Health," Fiber: Nutrition Source"

Heaton KW, Marcus SN, Emmett PH, Bolton DH (1988). "Particle Size Of Wheat, Maize, Oat Test Meals; Effects On Plasma Glucose And Insulin Responses And Rate Of Starch Digestion In Vitro" . Am J Clin Nutr. 47: 675–82.

Hellendoorn Ew 1983, "Fermentation As The Principal Cause Of The Physiological Activity Of Indigestible Food Residue." In: Spiller GA (ed) topics In Dietary Fiber Research. Plenum Press, New York, pp 127-168

Hermansson AM. "Gel Structure Of Food Biopolymers In: Food Structure, Its Creation And Evaluation" .JMV Blanshard and JR Mitchell, eds. 1988 pp. 25-40 Butterworths, London.

Institute of Medicine; Food and Nutrition Board. Dietary Reference Intakes: Energy, Carbohydrates, Fiber, Fat, Fatty Acids, Cholesterol, Protein And Amino Acids. Washington (DC): National Academies Press; 2005.

Jenkins DJ, Wolever TM, Leeds AR, et al. (1978). "Dietary Fibres, Fibre Analogues And Glucose Tolerance: Importance Of Viscosity". Br Med J. 1 (6124): 1392–94. doi:10.1136/bmj.1. 6124.1392.

Johnston, KL; Thomas EL; Bell JD; Frost GS; Robertson MD (April 2010). "Resistant Starch Improves Insulin Sensitivity In Metabolic Syndrome". Diabetic Medicine. 27 (4): 391–397. doi:10.1111/j.1464-5491. 2010. 02923.x. PMID 20536509.

James, S. "P208. "Abnormal Fibre Utilisation And Gut Transit In Ulcerative Colitis In Remission: A Potential New Target For Dietary Intervention". Presentation at European Crohn's & Colitis Organization meeting, Feb 16-18, 2012 in Barcelona, Spain. European Crohn's & Colitis Organization. Retrieved 25 September 2016.

Johnston, KL; Thomas EL; Bell JD; Frost GS; Robertson MD (2010). "Resistant Starch Improves Insulin Sensitivity In Metabolic Syndrome". Diabetic Medicine. 27 (4): 391–397. doi: 10.1111/j. 1464-5491.2010.02923.x. PMID 20536509.

Jones PJ, Varady KA (2008). "Are Functional Foods Redefining Nutritional Requirements?". Appl Physiol Nutr

Metab. 33 (1): 118–23. doi:10.1139/H07-134. PMID 18347661.Archived from the original (PDF) on 2012-02-27.

Kaur N, Gupta AK (December 2002). "Applications Of Inulin And Oligofructose In Health And Nutrition" (Pdf). J Biosci. 27 (7): 703–14. doi: 10.1007/BF02708379. PMID 12571376.

Keenan, M. J.; Martin, R. J.; Raggio, A. M.; McCutcheon, K. L.; Brown, I. L.; Birkett, A.; Newman, S. S.; Skaf, J.; Hegsted, M.; Tulley, R. T.; Blair, E.; Zhou, J. (2012). "High-Amylose Resistant Starch Increases Hormones And Improves Structure And Function Of The Gastrointestinal Tract: A Microarray Study". Journal of Nutrigenetics and Nutrigenomics. 5 (1):26–44. doi:10.1159/ 000335319. PMID 22516953.

Kevin, Maki; Pelkman CL; Finocchiaro ET; Kelley KM; Lawless AL; Schild AL; Rains TM (April 2012). "Resistant Starch From High-Amylose Maize Increases Insulin Sensitivity In Overweight And Obese Men". Journal of Nutrition. 142 (4): 717–723. doi: 10.3945/jn.111.152975. PMC 3301990. PMID 22357745

Liber, A.; Szajewska, H. (2013). "Effects Of Inulin-Type Fructans On Appetite, Energy Intake, And Body Weight In Children And Adults: Systematic Review Of Randomized Controlled Trials". Ann Nutr Metab. 63 (1–2): 42–54. doi:10.1159/ 000350312. PMID 23887189.

Linus Pauling Institute at Oregon State University

Lee YP, Puddey IB, Hodgson JM (April 2008). "Protein, Fiber And Blood Pressure: Potential Benefit Of Legumes". Clin Exp Pharmacol Physiol. 35 (4): 473–

6. doi:10.1111/j.1440-1681.2008. 04899.x. PMID 18307744.

Lustig RH (December 2006). "The 'Skinny' On Childhood Obesity: How Our Western Environment Starves Kids' Brains". Pediatr Ann. 35 (12): 898–902, 905–7. PMID 17236437.

Maki, Kevin C.; Pelkman CL; Finocchiaro ET; Kelley KM; Lawless AL; Schild AL; Rains TM (April 2012). "Resistant Starch From High-Amylose Maize Increases Insulin Sensitivity In Over-Weight And Obese Men". Journal of Nutrition. 142 (4): 717–723. doi:10.3945/ jn.111.152975. PMC 3301990. PMID 22357745.

MacDermott RP (January 2007). "Treatment Of Irritable Bowel Syndrome In Outpatients With Inflammatory Bowel Disease Using A Food And Beverage Intolerance, Food And Beverage Avoidance Diet". Inflamm Bowel Dis. 13 (1):91–6. doi:10.1002/ibd.20048. PMID 17206644.

MedlinePlus Medical Encyclopedia: Fiber. Retrieved 22 April 2009.

Nugent, Anne P (2005). "Health Properties Of Resistant Starch". nutrition Bulletin. 30 (1): 27–54. doi:10. 1111/ j.1467-3010.2005. 00481.x

Parisi GC, Zilli M, Miani MP, Carrara M, Bottona E, Verdianelli G, Battaglia G, Desideri S, Faedo A, Marzolino C, etal (2002). "High-fiber Diet Supplementation In Patients With Irritable Bowel Syndrome (IBS): A Multicenter, Randomized, Open Trial Comparison Between Wheat Bran Diet And Partially Hydrolyzed Guar Gum (PHGG)". dig Dis Sci. 47 (8): 1697–704. doi:10.1023/A: 1016419906546. PMID 12184518.

Park Y, Subar AF, Hollenbeck A, Schatzkin A (14 February 2011). "Dietary Fiber Intake And Mortality In The Nih-Aarp Diet And Health Study". Arch Intern Med. 171 (12): 1061–8. doi:10.1001/archinternmed. 2011.18. PMC 3513325. PMID 21321288.

Phillips, Jodi; Muir JG; Birkett A; Lu ZX; Jones GP; O'Dea K (July 1995). "Effect Of Resistant Starch On Fecal Bulk And Fermentation-Dependent Events In Humans". American Journal of Clinical Nutrition. 62 (1): 121–130.

Raghupathy, P; Ramakrishna BS; Oommen SP; Ahmed MS; Priyaa G; Dziura J; Young GP; Binder HJ (2006). "Amylase-resistant Starch As Adjunct To Oral Re-Hydration Therapy In Children With Diarrhea". Journal of Pediatric Gastro-enterology and Nutrition. 42 (4):362–368. doi:10.1097/01.mpg.0000214163. 83316.41. PMID 16641573.

Ramakrishna, BS; Venkataraman S; Srinivasan P; Dash P; Young GP; Binder HJ (February 2000). "Amylase-resistant Starch Plus Oral Rehydration Solution For Cholera". The New England Journal of Medicine. 342: 308–313. doi:10.1056/NEJM20000 2033420502. PMID 10655529.
Ramakrishna, Balakrishnan S.; Subramanian V; Mohan V; Sebastian BK; Young GP; Farthing MJ; Binder HJ (2008). "A Randomized Controlled Trial Of Glucose Versus Amylase Resistant Starch Hypo-Osmolar Oral Rehydration Solution For Adult Acute Dehydrating Diarrhea". PLoS ONE. 3 (2): e1587. Doi: 10. 1371/ journal. pone.0001587. PMC 2217593 . PMID 18270575.

Raschka L, Daniel H (November 2005). "Mechanisms Underlying The Effects Of Inulin-Type Fructans On

Calcium Absorption In The Large Intestine Of Rats". Bone. 37 (5): 728–35. doi:10. 1016/j. Bone.2005.05. 015. PMID 16126464.

Roberfroid MB (1 November 2007). "Inulin-type Fructans: Functional Food Ingredients". J Nutr. 137 (11 Suppl): 2493S–2502S. PMID 17951492.

Robertson, M. Denise; Currie JM; Morgan LM. Jewell DP; Frayn KN (2003). "Prior Short-Term Consumption Of Resistant Starch Enhances Postprandial Insulin Sensitivity In Healthy Subjects" (Pdf). diabetologia. 46 (5): 659–665. doi:10. 1007/s00125-003-1081-0. PMID 12712245.

Robertson, M. Denise; Bickerton AS; Dennis AL; Vidal H; Frayn KN (2005). "Insulin-sensitizing Effects Of Dietary Resistant Starch And Effects On Skeletal Muscle And Adipose Tissue Metabolism". The American Journal of Clinical Nutrition. 82 (3): 559–567. PMID 16155268.

Robertson, M. Denise; Wright JW; Loizon E; Debard C; Vidal H; Shojaee-Moradie F; Russell-Jones D; Umpleby AM (28 June 2012). "Insulin-sensitizing Effects On Muscle And Adipose Tissue After Dietary Fiber Intake In Men And Women With Metabolic Syndrome". Journal of Clinical Endocrinology & Meta-bolism. 97 (9):3326–32.doi: 10. 1210/jc.2012-1513. PMID 22745235.51

Rockland LB, Stewart GF. "Water Activity: Influences on Food Quality". Academic Press, New York. 1991

Rodríguez-Cabezas ME, Gálvez J, Camuesco D, et al. (October 2003). "Intestinal Anti-Inflammatory Activity Of Dietary Fiber (Plantago Ovata Seeds) In Hla-B27 Transgenic Rats". Clin Nutr. 22 (5):463–71. doi:10.1016/S0261-5614(03)00045-1. PMID 14512034.

Roy CC, Kien CL, Bouthillier L, Levy E (August 2006). "Short-chain Fatty Acids: Ready For Prime Time?". Nutr Clin Pract. 21 (4): 351–66. doi: 10. 1177/ 0115426506021004351. PMID 16870803.

Säemann MD, Böhmig GA, Zlabinger GJ (May 2002). "Short-chain Fatty Acids: Bacterial Mediators Of A Balanced Host-Microbial Relationship In The Human Gut". Wien Klin Wochenschr. 114 (8–9): 289–300. PMID 12212362.

Schatzkin A, Mouw T, Park Y, Subar AF, Kipnis V, Hollenbeck A, Leitzmann MF, Thompson FE (2007). "Dietary Fiber And Whole-Grain Consumption In Relation To Colorectal Cancer In The Nih-Aarp Diet And Health Study". Am J Clin Nutr. 85 (5): 1353–60. PMID 17490973.

Schneeman BO, Gallacher D. "Effects Of Dietary Fibre On Digestive Enzyme Activity And Bile Acids In The Small Intestine." Proc Soc Exp Biol Med 1985; 180 409-14.

Scholz-Ahrens KE, Ade P, Marten B, et al. (1 March 2007) . "Prebiotics, Pro-Biotics, And Synbiotics Affect Mineral Absorption, Bone Mineral Content, And Bone Structure". J Nutr. 137 (3 Suppl 2): 838S–46S. PMID 17311984.

Scholz-Ahrens KE, Schrezenmeir J (Nov 2007). "Inulin And Oligofructose And Mineral Metabolism: The Evidence From Animal Trials". J Nutr. 137 (11 Suppl): 2513S–2523S. PMID 17951495.

Seidner DL, Lashner BA, Brzezinski A, et al. (April 2005). "An Oral Supplement Enriched With Fish Oil, Soluble

Fiber, And Antioxidants For Corticosteroid Sparing In Ulcerative Colitis: A Randomized, Controlled Trial". Clin Gastroenterol Hepatol. 3 (4): 358–69. doi:10.1016/S1542-3565(04)00672-X. PMID 15822041.

Shepherd, Susan J.; Gibson, Peter R. (2006). "Fructose Malabsorption and Symptoms of Irritable Bowel Syndrome: Guidelines for Effective Dietary Management". Journal of the American Dietetic Association. 106 (10): 1631–1639. doi:10. 1016/j.jada. 2006.07.010. PMID 17000196.

Simons CCJM; et al. (October 2010). "Bowel Movement and Constipation Frequencies and the Risk of Colorectal Cancer Among Men in the Netherlands Cohort Study on Diet and Cancer". Am J Epidemiol. 172 (12): 1404–14. doi:10.1093/ aje/ kwq307. PMID 20980354.

Simpson, H. L.; Campbell, B. J. (2015). "Review Article: Dietary Fibre–Micro-Biota Interactions". Alimentary Pharma-cology & Therapeutics. 42 (2): 158–179. doi:10. 1111/ apt.13248. PMID 26011307.

Simpson, H; Campbell, BJ; Rhodes, JM (2014). "IBD: Microbiota Manipulation Through Diet And Modified Bacteria.". dig Dis. 32 Suppl1: 13–25. doi:10.1159/ 000367821.

Spiller, Gene; Margo N. Woods; Sherwood L. Gorbach (27 June 2001). Influence Of Fiber On The Ecology Of The Intestinal Flora. crc Handbook Of Dietary Fiber In Human Nutrition., crc Press. p. 257. ISBN 978-0-8493-2387-4. Retrieved 22 April 2009.

Stacewicz-Sapuntzakis M, Bowen PE, Hussain EA, Damayanti-Wood BI, Farnsworth NR (May 2001).

"Chemical Composition And Potential Health Effects Of Prunes: A Functional Food?". Crit Rev Food Sci Nutr. 41 (4):251–86. doi:10.1080/ 20014 091091814. PMID 11401245.

Suter PM (2005). "Carbohydrates And Dietary Fiber". Handb Exp Pharmacol. Handbook of Experimental Pharmacology. 170 (170):231–61. doi:10.1007/3-540-27661-0_8. ISBN 3-540-22569-2. PMID 16596802.

Tako E, Glahn RP, Welch RM, Lei X, Yasuda K, Miller DD (2007). "Dietary Inulin Affects The Expression Of Intestinal Enterocyte Iron Transporters, Receptors And Storage Protein And Alters The Microbiota In The Pig Intestine". Br J Nutr. 99 (Sep): 1–9. doi:10.1017/ S0007114507825128. PMID 17868492.

Theuwissen E, Mensink RP (May 2008). "Water-soluble Dietary Fibers And Cardiovascular Disease". Physiol. Behav. 94 (2): 285–92. doi:10.1016/ j. physbeh.2008. 01.001. PMID 18302966.

Tungland_Bc, Meyer D, "Nondigestible Oligo- And Poly-Saccharides (Dietary Fiber): Their Physiology And Role In Human Health And Food," Comp Rev Food Sci Food Safety, 3:73-92, 2002 (Table 3)[1]

United Kingdom, "The Food Labeling Regulations 1996 – Schedule 7: Nutrition Labeling"

USDA, "National Nutrient Database for Standard Reference, Release 17, Fiber Data "

USDA; Agricultural Research Service. "What We Eat In America: Nutrient Intakes From Food By Gender And Age." National Health and Nutrition Examination Survey

(NHANES) 2007–2008 [cited 2012 Feb 20] www.ars.usda.gov/SP2UserFiles/Place/ 12355000/ pdf/ 0708 /Table_1_NIN_GEN_ 07. pdf

US Department of Agriculture, National Agricultural Library and National Academy of Sciences, Institute of Medicine, Food and Nutrition Board, "Dietary Reference Intakes For Energy, Carbohydrate, Fibre, Fat, Fatty Acids, Cholesterol, Protein, And Amino Acids (Macronutrients) (2005), "Chapter 7: Dietary, Functional and Total fibre" (PDF).

U.S. Government Printing Office, "Soluble Fiber from Certain Foods and Risk of Coronary Heart Disease,, Electronic Code of Federal Regulations," Title 21: Food and Drugs, part 101: Food Labeling, Subpart E, Specific Requirements for Health Claims, 101.81 [2]

U.S. Government Printing Office, Electronic Code Of Federal Regulations, Health Claims: Fiber-Containing Grain Products, Fruits, And Vegetables And Cancer. Current As Of 20 October 2008

U.S. Government Printing Office, "Health Claims: Fruits, Vegetables, And Grain Products That Contain Fiber, Particularly Soluble Fiber, And Risk Of Coronary Heart Disease". Electronic Code of Federal Regulations: current as of 20 October 2008

University of MD Medical Center Encyclopedia entry for "Fiber". Retrieved 22 April 2009.

Venn BJ, Mann JI (November 2004). "Cereal Grains, Legumes And Diabetes". eur J Clin Nutr. 58 (11):1443–61. doi:10.1038/ sj. Ejcn. 1601995. PMID 15162131.

Ward PB, Young GP (1997). "Dynamics Of Clostridium Difficile Infection. Control Using Diet". Adv Exp Med Biol. 412: 63–75. PMID 9191992.

WebMD-- Constipation

WebMD--/vitamins--supplements,Konjac+glucomannan

Weickert MO, Pfeiffer AF (2008). "Metabolic Effects Of Dietary Fiber Consumption And Prevention Of Diabetes". J Nutr. 138 (3): 439–42. PMID 18287346.

Wong JM, de Souza R, Kendall CW, Emam A, Jenkins DJ (March 2006). "Colonic Health: Fermentation And Short Chain Fatty Acids". J Clin Gastroenterol. 40 (3):235–43. doi:10.1097/ 0000 4836-200603000-00015. PMID 16633129.

Zhang, Wen-qing; Wang Hong-wei; Zhang Yue-ming; Yang Yue-xin (March 2007). "Effects Of Resistant Starch On Insulin Resistance Of Type 2 Diabetes Mellitus Patients". Chinese Journal of Preventive Medicine. 41 (2): 101–104. PMID 17605234.

www.ingramcontent.com/pod-product-compliance
Lightning Source LLC
Chambersburg PA
CBHW070044210526
45170CB00012B/577